Complications in Orthopaedics
Tibial Shaft Fractures

Edited by
William M. Ricci, MD
Assistant Professor
Department of Orthopaedics
Washington University School of Medicine
St. Louis, Missouri

Series Editor
Jeffrey O. Anglen, MD
Boone Orthopaedic Associates
Columbia, Missouri

Published by the
American Academy of Orthopaedic Surgeons
6300 North River Road
Rosemont, IL 60018

American Academy of Orthopaedic Surgeons

American Academy of Orthopaedic Surgeons
6300 North River Road
Rosemont, IL 60018
1-800-626-6726

The material presented in *Tibial Shaft Fractures* has been made available by the American Academy of Orthopaedic Surgeons for educational purposes only. This material is not intended to present the only, or necessarily best, methods or procedures for the medical situations discussed, but rather is intended to represent an approach, view, statement, or opinion of the author(s) or producer(s), which may be helpful to others who face similar situations.

Some drugs or medical devices demonstrated in Academy courses or described in Academy print or electronic publications have not been cleared by the Food and Drug Administration (FDA) or have been cleared for specific uses only. The FDA has stated that it is the responsibility of the physician to determine the FDA clearance status of each drug or device he or she wishes to use in clinical practice.

PMMA bone cement is considered a device for FDA purposes. In October 1999, the FDA reclassified PMMA bone cement as a Class II device for its intended use "in arthroplastic procedures of the hip, knee, and other joints for the fixation of polymer or metallic prosthetic implants to living bone." The use of a device for other than its FDA-cleared indication is an off-label use. Physicians may use a device off-label if they believe, in their best medical judgment, that its use is appropriate for a particular patient (eg, tumors).

Furthermore, any statements about commercial products are solely the opinion(s) of the author(s) and do not represent an Academy endorsement or evaluation of these products. These statements may not be used in advertising or for any commercial purpose.

First Edition

ISBN 0-89203-330-4

Bone and Joint DECADE 2002 - USA - 2011

Contributors

Joseph Borelli, Jr, MD
Associate Professor
Chief, Orthopaedic Trauma Service
Department of Orthopaedics
Washington University School of Medicine
St. Louis, Missouri

William M. Ricci, MD
Assistant Professor
Department of Orthopaedics
Washington University School of Medicine
St. Louis, Missouri

Contents

Preface

The tibia is the most common site of long bone fractures in adults. Although tibial shaft fractures heal uneventfully in most patients, this injury has a much higher rate of complications compared with other long bone fractures. Multiple factors contribute to these complications; some specific to the tibia (and its inherent healing capacity), some to the associated soft-tissue injury, and others attributable to technical difficulty in applying a specific treatment modality.

The most common complications associated with tibia fractures include nonunion, delayed union, malalignment, infection, and pain. Avoiding these complications requires well-planned initial fracture and soft-tissue management and close clinical observation during the postinjury and postoperative periods. Even with optimal treatment planning and execution, complications may occur. Timely recognition and management may enable salvage and, ultimately, an acceptable result.

In this first volume of this new series of case-based monographs that focuses on recognition, management, and ultimately potential avoidance of common complications in orthopaedics, problems associated with tibial shaft fractures are most appropriately the first to be addressed. The first section of each chapter is the case presentation, which consists of the history, physical examination, radiographic findings of initial injury, and a brief description of the initial treatment and follow-up to the point at which a complication requiring treatment is recognized. At this point in each chapter, the reader may wish to pause and reflect on how he or she would approach and treat the patient and the problem in his/her own practice. The second section of each chapter is a discussion of the problem, including details on how to recognize it, identify situations at potentially high risk, manage the complication, and finally create strategies to avoid the particular complication. The final section of each chapter revisits the original case, summarizing the method and rationale selected to manage the particular complication, and its ultimate outcome. The individual sections deal specifically with compartment syndrome, malalignment after IM nailing, acute infection, malunion, aseptic nonunion, infected nonunion, chronic knee and implant-related pain, and failure of nonunion repair.

The surgeon cannot influence the inherent healing capacity of the tibia, the comorbidities of the patient, or the severity of the bone and soft-tissue injury. However, we must understand these issues and apply the most appropriate treatment modality to maximize healing potential and minimize associated complications. This volume offers insight for the practicing orthopaedic surgeon to avoid or manage common preoperative, intraoperative, and postoperative complications encountered while treating tibial shaft fractures.

For this project to progress from concept to print, many people devoted significant time and resources. I thank Dr. Jeffrey Anglen, Series Editor, for his guidance in selecting and preparing topics for this volume; Karen O'Dell, my secretary, for her many hours of dedicated and skillful work revising the following chapters; Lynne Shindoll, Managing Editor, for her untiring editorial efforts; the AAOS Publications Committee for their commitment to this new series; Dr. Joseph Borrelli, my partner and friend, for his contributions to this volume; and most importantly Ann, Michael, and Luke, my family, for their patience and support during the many hours that I spent time away from them so that I could prepare this volume.

William M. Ricci, MD
Editor

Chapter 1

Compartment Syndrome

William M. Ricci, MD

Case Presentation

History

A 25-year-old man sustained closed midshaft tibia and fibula fractures after he was kicked while playing soccer. Upon arrival at the emergency department, he reported right lower extremity pain, deformity, and swelling. His medical history was insignificant, and he did not use tobacco. In addition, he did not have diabetes mellitus.

On initial examination, he appeared to be a well-developed, well-nourished athletic man. The right lower extremity had mild swelling, ecchymosis, tenderness and deformity. Pulses were present and equal on the left side, sensation was intact, and all compartments were soft. **Figure 1** shows his initial AP and lateral radiographs. Based on his clinical presentation and radiographs, an initial diagnosis of closed displaced midshaft tibia and fibula fractures was made.

Initial Management

In the emergency department, the patient was placed in a long leg splint and admitted to the hospital. The following day he underwent uncomplicated reamed intramedullary nailing under general anesthesia. A tourniquet was used until the reaming process, and then released for the remainder of the procedure. Reaming was performed up to 11 mm at 0.5-mm increments and a 10-mm nail was inserted. Chatter was encountered with the 10.5-mm reamer. Intraoperative radiographs confirmed satisfactory fracture reduction, limb alignment, and position of the intramedullary device and interlocking bolts (**Figure 2**). The patient was placed in a short leg splint postoperatively for comfort.

Postoperatively the patient had intravenous morphine patient-controlled analgesia (PCA) for 36 hours and then was converted to oral analgesia. On the first postoperative day, the patient reported mild to moderate pain that was well controlled with the PCA morphine. Sensation distally was intact, and capillary refill was good. On the morning of postoperative day 2, the patient stated that he was comfortable, but he reported that he had significantly increased pain overnight. On examination, he had decreased sensation on the dorsum of the foot, minimal pain with passive range of motion of the ankle and toes, good pulses, and good capillary refill. The new-onset paresthesias combined with a history of increased pain over the previous 8 hours suggested a potential com-

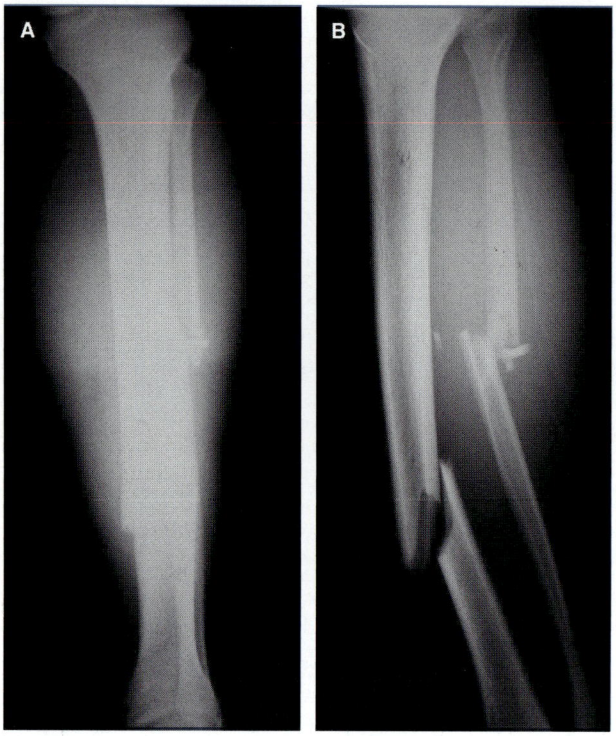

Figure 1 AP (**A**) and lateral (**B**) radiographs of the injury.

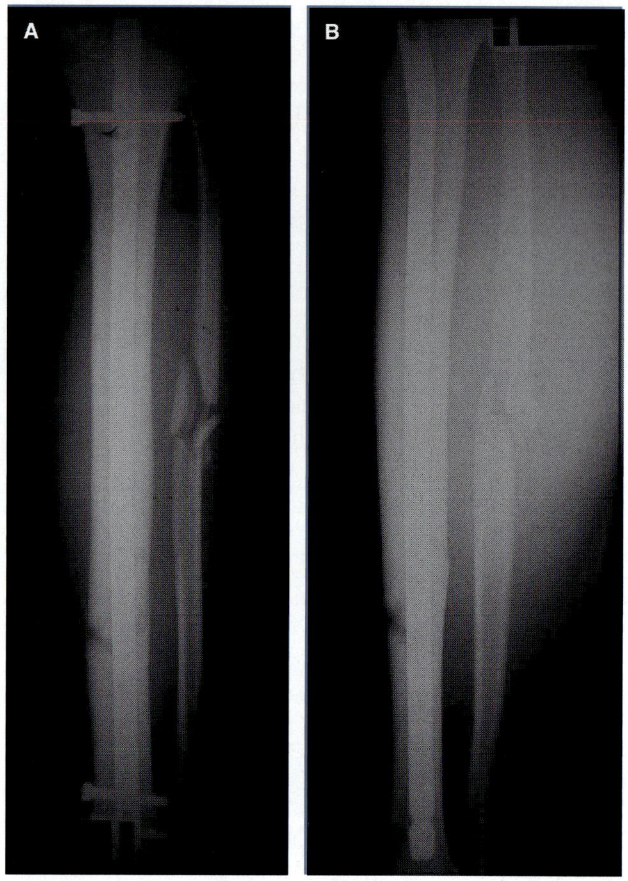

Figure 2 AP (**A**) and lateral (**B**) radiographs after the index nailing procedure.

partment syndrome. The splint was removed and the compartments examined. Hard anterior and lateral compartments and a relatively soft posterior compartment were found. Compartment syndrome was diagnosed clinically, and the patient was brought emergently to the operating room for fasciotomy.

Fasciotomy of the anterior and lateral compartments was performed through a single lateral incision. The anterior compartment musculature was found to be of poor color, consistency, and contractility in a 10- to 12-cm central zone. The proximal muscle appeared to be viable. The lateral compartment musculature appeared to be of normal color, consistency, and contractility. A fasciotomy of the posterior compartment was not performed. The wound was packed open.

Status of Complication

The patient had an unrecognized compartment syndrome. Fasciotomy revealed a 10- to 12-cm zone of nonviable anterior compartment musculature. The patient was then transferred to a tertiary care facility for further management. The lateral fasciotomy wound remained open. The patient had decreased sensation over the entire dorsum of the foot and in the first web space. Strength of the tibialis anterior muscle was 0/5, the extensor hallucis longus was 0/5, and the extensor digitorum was 2/5. Peroneal strength was 3/5, and the ankle and toe flexors were 4/5.

Discussion

Recognizing the Problem and Situations at High Risk

Compartment syndrome is characterized by elevated tissue pressures within a closed myofascial compartment that reduce capillary perfusion below a level necessary to maintain tissue viability.[1] This lack of perfusion causes ischemia to the components of the compartment, of which the muscles and nerves are most sensitive. Untreated, this ischemia leads to necrosis, followed by fibrosis of the affected structures with associated functional and sensory deficit. Fracture, vascular injury, overexertion, prolonged compression, burns, and even minor trauma (in anticoagulated patients) can cause compartment syndrome.

Fracture, the most common cause, results in increased compartment pressure from edema and hemorrhage, which leads to venous obstruction, closure of arterioles, and eventual muscle and nerve ischemia.

Patients who sustain high-energy injuries, have hypotension, take anticoagulants, or who have excessively tight dressings or casts are at increased risk. Patients with open fractures are not free of risk, as the incidence of compartment syndrome in open tibia fractures has been reported to be 9%, with the risk proportional to the degree of injury to soft tissue and bone.[2]

Diagnosing Compartment Syndrome

Compartment syndrome is primarily a clinical diagnosis. The hallmarks of compartment syndrome include the so-called six "Ps": pain, paresthesias, pressure, paralysis, pallor, and pulselessness. Pain is a relatively early sign; its severity is usually out of proportion to the injury, often occurs with passive stretch of muscles in the involved compartment, and is not relieved with usual doses of narcotic analgesia. Paresthesias usually include numbness and tingling but are often poorly defined and poorly localized. Pressure manifests itself as a tense compartment on physical examination. Deep compartments cannot be accurately evaluated; therefore, lack of a tense compartment is not an accurate sign. Paralysis involves the inability to actively move the muscles within the involved compartment. Pallor indicates poor tissue profusion distal to the area of increased pressure. Pulselessness occurs in the very late stage of compartment syndrome when the tissue pressure is greater than the systolic blood pressure. A diagnosis should be made when the tissue pressure is approximately 50 mm Hg, well below the pressure required to produce pulselessness.

Compartment pressure measurements are not mandatory but can be used as an adjunct to clinical diagnosis. These measurements are especially useful to rule out compartment syndrome rather than to confirm its presence. A compartment pressure within 30 mm of Hg of the diastolic blood pressure confirms a compartment syndrome.[3] Absolute measurements of compartment pressure have been advocated but are less reliable.[4,5] In patients who are hypotensive, an absolute pressure threshold may cause the diagnosis to be missed inadvertently. Conversely, in patients with hypertension, an absolute pressure threshold may result in an inaccurate positive diagnosis and lead to unnecessary fasciotomy. When obtaining pressure measurements, all four compartments of the leg should be assessed at the level of, and at varying distances from, the fracture because compartment pressures have been shown to have a gradient surrounding the zone of injury.[6]

Patients with altered mental status as a result of the injury or from intoxication require especially careful observation and monitoring because clinical signs of compartment syndrome are unreliable. Indwelling, continuous compartment pressure measurements have been advocated for these patients. The latter approach is more popular in Europe where even alert, oriented patients sometimes are continuously monitored. Patients should be monitored preoperatively and at least 24 hours postoperatively, but the precise duration of monitoring that is necessary remains unclear.

Management of Compartment Syndrome

Once a diagnosis of compartment syndrome is made, either clinically or with compartment pressure measurement, emergent fasciotomy is indicated. Irreversible muscle necrosis occurs after approximately 4 to 8 hours of ischemia, and irreversible nerve injury occurs after approximately 8 to 12 hours of ischemia.

Once the diagnosis is confirmed, all four compartments should be addressed. The deep posterior and anterior compartments are the most commonly involved. In general, all four compartments should be fasciotomized. Occasionally, one compartment is obviously involved and after fasciotomy of this compartment, the others are found to be soft. Fasciotomy of the uninvolved compartments can be deferred only after confirmation of normal compartment pressures. These patients must continue to be closely monitored for compartment syndrome of the nonfasciotomized compartments.

One incision and two incision techniques can be used.[7] I advocate the two-incision technique, which includes a lateral incision, centered between the fibula and the crest of the tibia. Through this incision, both anterior and lateral compartments can be addressed. Great care must be taken to avoid injury of the superficial peroneal nerve as it exits the lateral compartment fascia. Distal fasciotomy should be done under direct visualization to avoid this complication. A posterior-medial incision is used to address both the superficial and deep posterior compartments. This incision is located just posterior to the posterior margin of the medial tibia, with care to avoid injury to the saphenous nerve and vein. The superficial compartment is directly exposed, and the deep compartment is accessed via careful dissection posterior to the tibia.

A single-incision technique has been advocated by some and includes a lateral incision at the level of the fibula, several centimeters more posterior than the lateral incision used for a two-incision technique. The superficial posterior compartment is exposed with subcutaneous dissection. Dissection posterior to the fibula through the fascia between the soleus and the flexor hallucis longus allows access to the deep posterior compartment. Anterior subcutaneous dissection allows exposure of the anterior and lateral compartments.[7]

After fasciotomy, all muscles of each compartment should be carefully examined for viability. Evaluation of contractility with Bovie stimulation, color, and consistency is required to assess the viability of the muscle. Nonviable muscle should be débrided. With any amount of nonviable muscle, repeat irrigation and débridement at 24- to 48-hour intervals are indicated until all remaining muscle is viable. The skin should be left open or loosely approximated between serial irrigation and débridement procedures. Once the muscle bed is clean and healthy, delayed primary skin closure (if without tension) or split-thickness skin graft of the area is indicated. Secondary excision of the skin graft and primary closure of the native skin can sometimes be performed at a later date for cosmesis.

When the entire muscle belly is found to be necrotic (as in the case of this patient), which is usually seen in the context of late or missed diagnosis, the fate of the muscle is controversial. Excision of the entire muscle belly permanently eliminates function of that muscle. When the proximal muscle remains viable, leaving the musculotendinous unit intact offers some hope of function but increases the risk of infection. This "trade off" can be of concern, especially when the involved muscles are adjacent to the fractured bone. In such instances, treatment with local wound care, such as a wound vacuum-controlled assisted closure (VAC) device, until a bed of healthy granulation tissue grows over the affect area is indicated until a skin graft can be applied over this granulation tissue. If any sign of infection develops, the entire zone of nonviable muscle should be completely débrided.

Preventing Compartment Syndrome

The severity of the soft-tissue and bone injury at the initial time of trauma is the most influential factor in the potential development of compartment syndrome. Surgeons have little control over injury severity. However, it is critical to avoid further soft-tissue trauma during both evaluation and treatment. Expeditious and careful immobilization in a long leg splint will help reduce soft-tissue trauma. Avoiding excessive fracture manipulation during all phases of the operative procedure, including prepping, draping, and stabilization, is crucial. Tight dressings, splints, and casts also should be avoided. Casts have been shown to decrease the volume allowed for tissue swelling, which can potentially increase compartment pressures. Elevation should be at the level of the heart. Excessive elevation should be avoided in patients at particular risk because it lowers venous pressure, thereby decreasing the threshold for compartment syndrome.

An appropriate index of suspicion, coupled with adequately educating the patient and the allied health personnel caring for the patient, is critical. Certainly, the physician cannot continuously monitor the patient. Therefore, educating the patient and the nursing staff about the risks and early signs of compartment syndrome is important. Any patient who reports increasingly severe pain that is out of proportion to the injury or pain that is not relieved with usual doses of narcotic analgesia should be evaluated by a physician for compartment syndrome.

Case Management and Outcome Summary

In this case, the early signs of compartment syndrome were not recognized. The segmental necrosis of the anterior compartment musculature presents an unusual and unfortunate problem. In this patient, the musculotendinous unit was left intact, despite the increased risk of infection.

The wound was treated with a wound VAC device for 2 weeks after which time granulation tissue formed abundantly over clearly viable muscle but more slowly over nonviable tissues (**Figure 3**). A split-thickness skin graft was applied and approximately 80% of the graft healed successfully. The additional area required prolonged local wound care but eventually healed (**Figure 4**). The fracture healed uneventfully (**Figure 5**), and he regained some ankle and toe dorsiflexion.

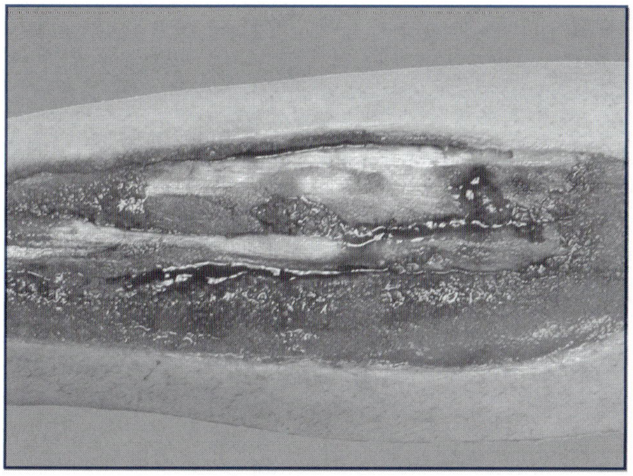

Figure 3 Clinical photograph showing early granulation tissue after placement of the VAC device.

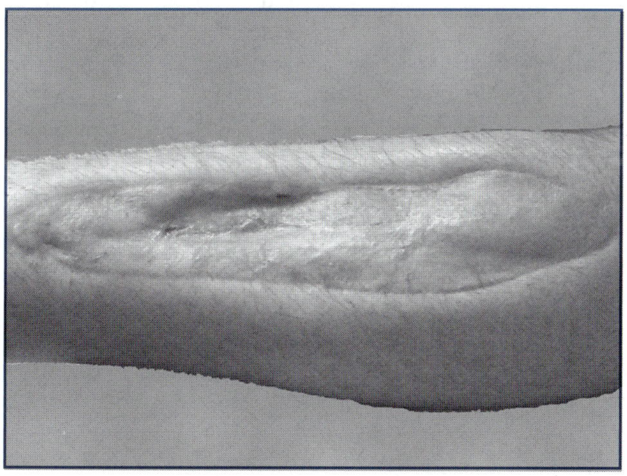

Figure 4 Clinical photograph showing the wound after skin grafting.

Strategies to Minimize Common Complications

A compartment syndrome is a potentially devastating problem if not recognized early and treated appropriately. In this case, if the patient was properly educated about the early signs of compartment syndrome, he may have been more diligent in notifying nursing staff of the increased pain he experienced overnight. Advising both the patient and the allied health staff caring for the patient about the risks and signs of compartment syndrome is helpful to avoid an unrecognized compartment syndrome.

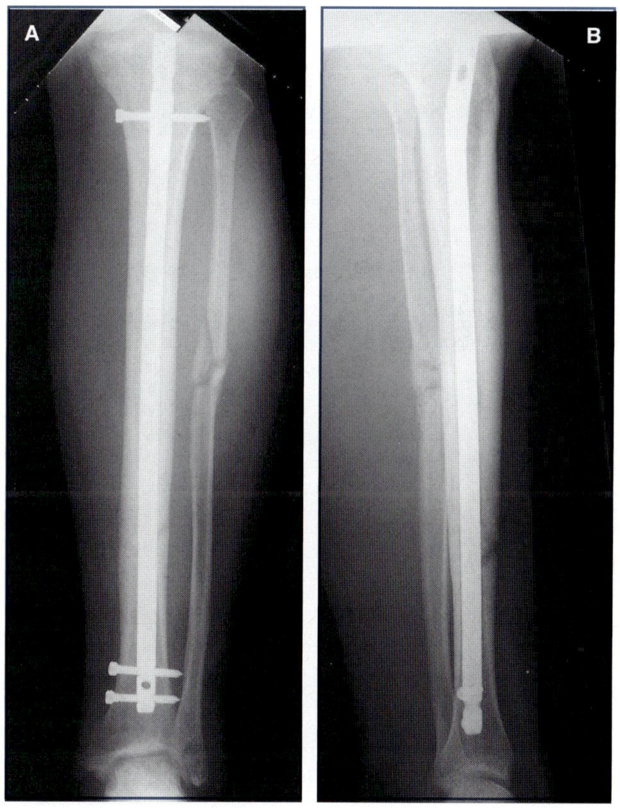

Figure 5 AP (**A**) and lateral (**B**) radiographs showing the healed fracture.

REFERENCES

1. Mubarak SJ, Hargens AR: *Compartment Syndrome and Volkman's Contracture.* Philadelphia, PA, WB Saunders, 1981.
2. Blick S, Brumback R, Poka A, Burgess A, Ebraheim NA: Compartment syndrome in open tibial fractures. *J Bone Joint Surg Am* 1986;68:1348-1353.
3. McQueen MM, Court BC: Compartment monitoring in tibial fractures: The pressure threshold for decompression. *J Bone Joint Surg Br* 1996;78:99-104.
4. Matsen FAI, Winquist RA, Krugmire RB: Diagnosis and management of compartment syndromes. *J Bone Joint Surg Am* 1980;62:286-291.
5. Whitesides TE, Haney TC, Morimoto K, Hirada H: Tissue pressure measurements as a determinant for the need of fasciotomy. *Clin Orthop* 1975;113:43.
6. Heckman MM, Whitesides TE Jr, Grewe SR, Rooks MD: Compartment pressure in association with closed tibial fractures: The relationship between tissue pressure, compartment, and the distance from the site of the fracture. *J Bone Joint Surg Am* 1994;76:1285-1292.
7. Heppenstall RB: Compartment syndrome: Pathophysiology, diagnosis, and treatment. *Tech Orthop* 1997;12:92-108.

Chapter 2

Malalignment

William M. Ricci, MD

Case Presentation

History

A 37-year-old pedestrian was struck by a motor vehicle traveling at approximately 30 miles per hour. He was transported by to the emergency department via emergency medical services with right lower extremity pain, deformity, and bleeding. He was otherwise healthy, did not smoke, did not have diabetes mellitus, and had no previous injuries to the right lower extremity. Physical examination in the emergency department revealed a 2-cm, bleeding longitudinal wound over the medial pretibial region of the proximal one third of leg with exposed tibia, swelling, and a valgus deformity. Pulses were palpable and equal to the contralateral side, and sensation was intact. There was no evidence of an acute compartment syndrome. The contralateral lower extremity was normal, and the patient had no other injuries or abnormalities. Initial radiographs revealed an oblique fracture involving the proximal one third of the tibial shaft and an associated comminuted fracture of the proximal fibula (**Figure 1**). No other abnormalities were noted. The initial diagnosis was open grade II fractures of the proximal tibia and fibula.

Initial Management

The patient was taken emergently to surgery for irrigation and débridement of the open fracture and intramedullary (IM) nailing of the tibia. The fracture was thoroughly débrided by removing devitalized soft tissue and bone. The wound was irrigated with 9 L of normal saline solution using pulsatile irrigation. IM nailing was performed through a medial parapatellar approach. The fracture was manually reduced during reaming and nailing. The nail was locked proximally and distally, and then the open wound closed definitively.

Status of Complication

Immediate postoperative radiographs revealed valgus malalignment after IM nailing of the proximal tibia fracture (**Figure 2**).

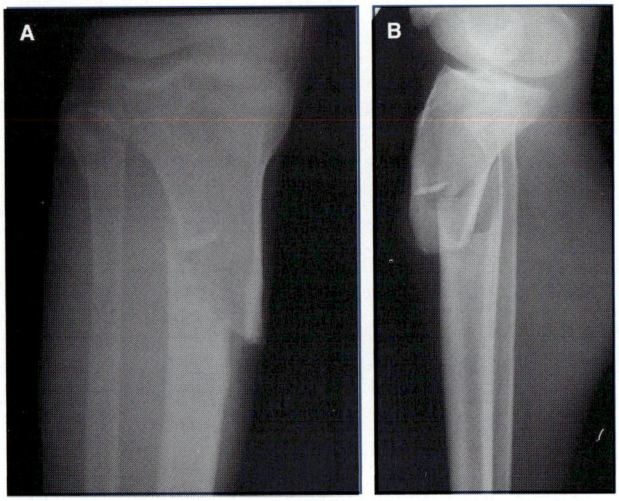

Figure 1 AP (**A**) and lateral (**B**) radiographs showing an oblique fracture of the proximal one third of the tibial shaft.

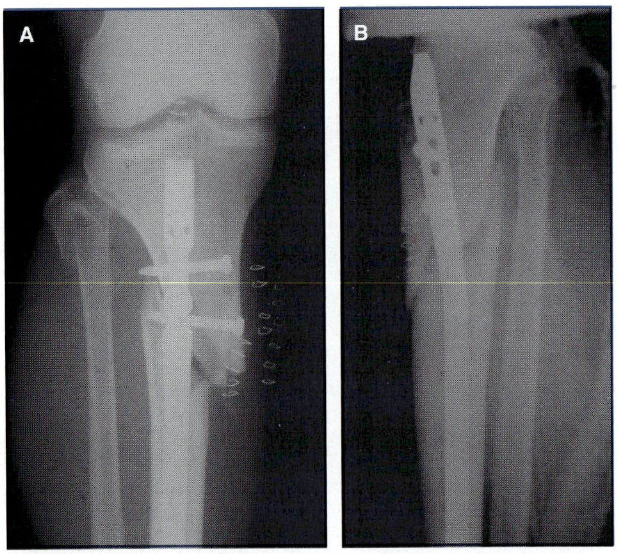

Figure 2 Postoperative AP (**A**) and lateral (**B**) radiographs showing valgus malalignment.

Discussion

Recognizing the Problem and Situations at High Risk

The incidence of malalignment following IM nailing is highly dependent on both fracture location and fracture pattern.[1] Fractures in the midshaft region, especially in proximity to the isthmus, are least prone to malalignment. The narrow canal in this region facilitates proper alignment of the IM nail within the proximal and distal fracture fragments in both the coronal and sagittal planes. Fractures of the proximal and distal thirds of the tibial shaft are most prone to malalignment due, in part, to the wide intramedullary space in these regions.

The increased potential for malalignment in fractures of the proximal shaft is related to the local anatomy, the fracture pattern, or technical factors. The intramedullary space is especially wide in this region. The strong forces exerted by the extensor mechanism have a propensity to cause apex anterior malalignment. The forces exerted by the anterior and lateral compartment musculature can contribute to valgus malalignment in this region. The obliquity of the fracture can also be a complicating factor. When the proximal fragment has a short or comminuted posterior segment, the nail is more likely to exit posteriorly in the proximal fragment, increasing the risk of apex anterior angulation (**Figure 3**, *A*). Similarly, when the proximal fragment has a short or comminuted lateral segment, the nail is more likely to exit posteriorly in the proximal fragment, increasing the risk of valgus malalignment (**Figure 3**, *B*).

Technical factors at the time of surgery also can contribute to deformity. A medial starting point and a laterally directed angle of insertion can lead to valgus malalignment.[1-3] A distal starting point and the "wedge effect" of a bent nail in the distal fragment can contribute to apex anterior malalignment.[2,4] Therefore, the surgeon must closely evaluate the fracture pattern of proximal tibia fractures, paying particular attention to obliquity and fracture comminution. In these cases, the preoperative plan should include contingencies for obtaining proper alignment.

Fractures of the distal shaft can also be problematic. The isthmus aligns the nail within the proximal fracture fragment in these cases; therefore, the position of the nail in the distal fracture fragment is of key importance for proper alignment. The location, presence, or absence of an associated fibula fracture can influence the frequency and direction of associated tibial malalignment after IM nailing. With an intact distal fibular segment, varus malalignment is the common deformity. With an associated fibula fracture at or near the level of the tibia fracture, the direction of malalignment is less predictable.

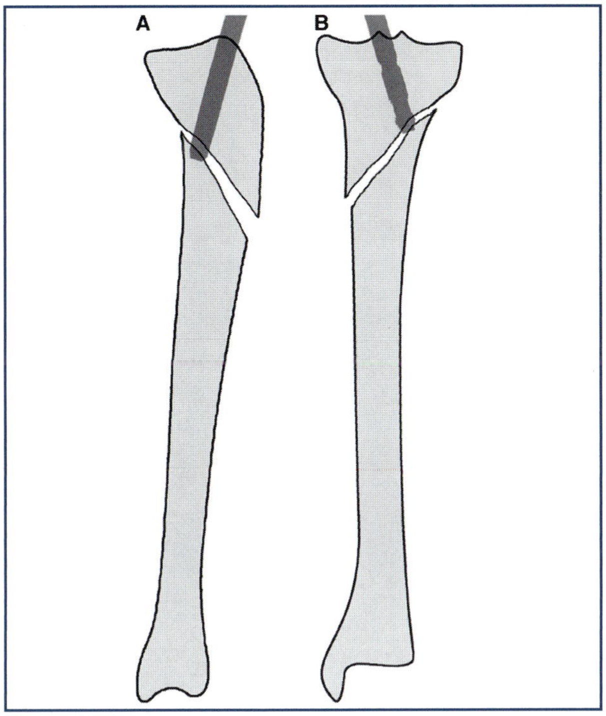

Figure 3 A, Diagram showing the nail exiting posteriorly in a short oblique proximal fragment. **B,** Diagram showing the nail exiting laterally in a short oblique proximal fragment.

The key to recognizing the potential for malalignment of end-segment tibial shaft fractures is the location and pattern of the fracture. However, only careful attention to surgical technique can prevent the complication. A thorough preoperative plan includes contingencies for the inability to obtain proper alignment with standard fixation techniques.

Managing Malalignment of Tibial Shaft Fractures

Management is best initiated by first recognizing the potential for the problem and careful preoperative planning and concludes with meticulous surgical technique.

Malalignment of proximal and distal tibial shaft fractures after IM nailing has been widely reported.[1,3,5,6] Freedman and Johnson[1] reported that the rate of malalignment was significantly higher in fractures of the proximal third than with fractures of either the middle or distal third in a retrospective review of 133 tibia fractures treated with IM nailing. In a different retrospective review of 32 proximal third tibia fractures treated with IM nailing, Lang and associates[3] reported that 84% of their patients had at least 5° of angulation, with valgus malalignment the most common problem.

I believe that blocking screws are the most reliable way to avoid malalignment when nailing proximal and distal tibia shaft fractures. Krettek and associates[7] described the use of blocking screws to supplement IM fixation of metaphyseal fractures. Blocking screws can be used to help obtain satisfactory alignment[8] and improve stability[9] during IM nailing of the tibia. This technique can be applied to any long bone fracture involving a metaphyseal region. Blocking screws are used to guide IM nails into the desired pathway. With proximal tibial shaft fractures, which are the most common application of this technique, blocking screws are placed into the distal portion of the proximal fracture fragment before nail insertion. The orientation and location of the screw(s) depends on the desired effect. To prevent apex anterior angulation, a blocking screw(s) is placed just posterior to the central axis of the tibia. The nail is then inserted anterior to the blocking screw, properly aligning it with the long axis of the proximal fragment in the sagittal plane (**Figure 4**). To prevent valgus angulation, a blocking screw(s) is placed just lateral to the central axis. The nail is inserted medial to the blocking screw, properly aligning it with the long axis in the coronal plane (**Figure 5**). As the nail is passed across the fracture, the isthmus serves to properly align the nail in the distal fragment (Figures 4 and 5). We reported that use of this technique on 12 consecutive patients with proximal one third tibia fractures resulted in less than 5° of angular deformity in all patients.[8]

Several other technical modifications to standard IM nailing technique can result in anatomic reduction. (1) Nailing with the knee in a semiextended position, combined with knee arthrotomy and lateral subluxation of the patella, has been successful in avoiding apex anterior angulation. In their report on 25 consecutive patients with proximal tibia fractures, Tornetta and Collins[10] reported that use of this technique resulted in a flexion deformity of only 5° or less in all of their patients. Disadvantages of this approach, however, are the requirement for a knee arthrotomy and the inability to address varus-valgus angulation. (2) Nailing with the knee in hyperflexion can help avoid apex anterior angulation by allowing an insertion angle parallel to the anterior cortex of the proximal fragment.[2] However, with

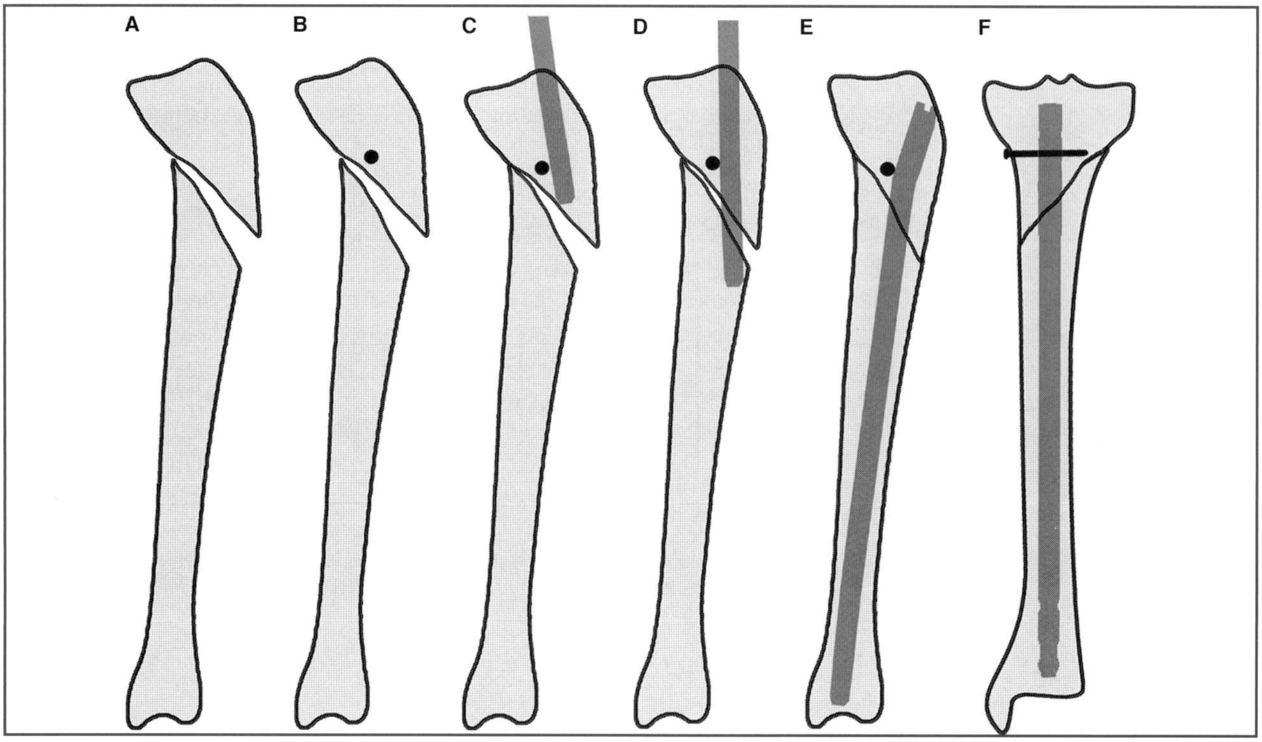

Figure 4 A posterior blocking screw helps prevent apex anterior angulation. **A,** Lateral view of a short oblique proximal third tibia fracture. **B,** A blocking screw is placed just posterior to the central axis in a medial-to-lateral direction. **C,** The nail is passed anterior to the blocking screw. **D,** The apex anterior angulation begins to be corrected as the nail is passed across the fracture site. **E,** The fracture is properly reduced after the nail is inserted completely. **F,** AP view of the tibia following insertion of the nail and blocking screw.

the knee in hyperflexion, the extensor mechanism is especially tight, and obtaining a proper insertion angle in the coronal plane becomes more difficult. (3) The use of a femoral distractor has also been advocated to neutralize the deforming muscle forces at the fracture site and to maintain anatomic reduction during nailing.[2] Half pins are placed through medial percutaneous wounds, one each in the proximal posterior metaphysis and in the distal posterior metaphysis to avoid interfering with nail placement. To help obtain neutral varus-valgus alignment, each pin is placed parallel to the articular surface (**Figure 6,** *A*). If pins are properly placed, a distracter applied between the pins will yield proper varus-valgus alignment (**Figure 6,** *B*).

Several other adjuncts can be used to help achieve proper alignment. Pointed reduction clamps placed percutaneously are especially useful for spiral and oblique midshaft fractures. Temporary short plates with unicortical screws can be placed across the fracture site through limited surgical incisions or open wounds. These screws should be removed after nailing to avoid mixing modes of fracture stabilization. Regardless of the method chosen, when using a guide wire for nailing, the guide wire must be aligned within both the proximal and distal fracture fragments before reaming and nail placement. Proper reaming technique requires that the fracture be reduced as the reamers are placed across the fracture. Any maneuvers used to achieve reduction as the guide wire is inserted should, therefore, be reproduced during the reaming process to avoid asymmetric reaming. Because the nail will follow the tract created during reaming, maintaining fracture alignment during reaming is critical to achieve proper alignment after nail placement.

Although IM nailing is the preferred treatment for

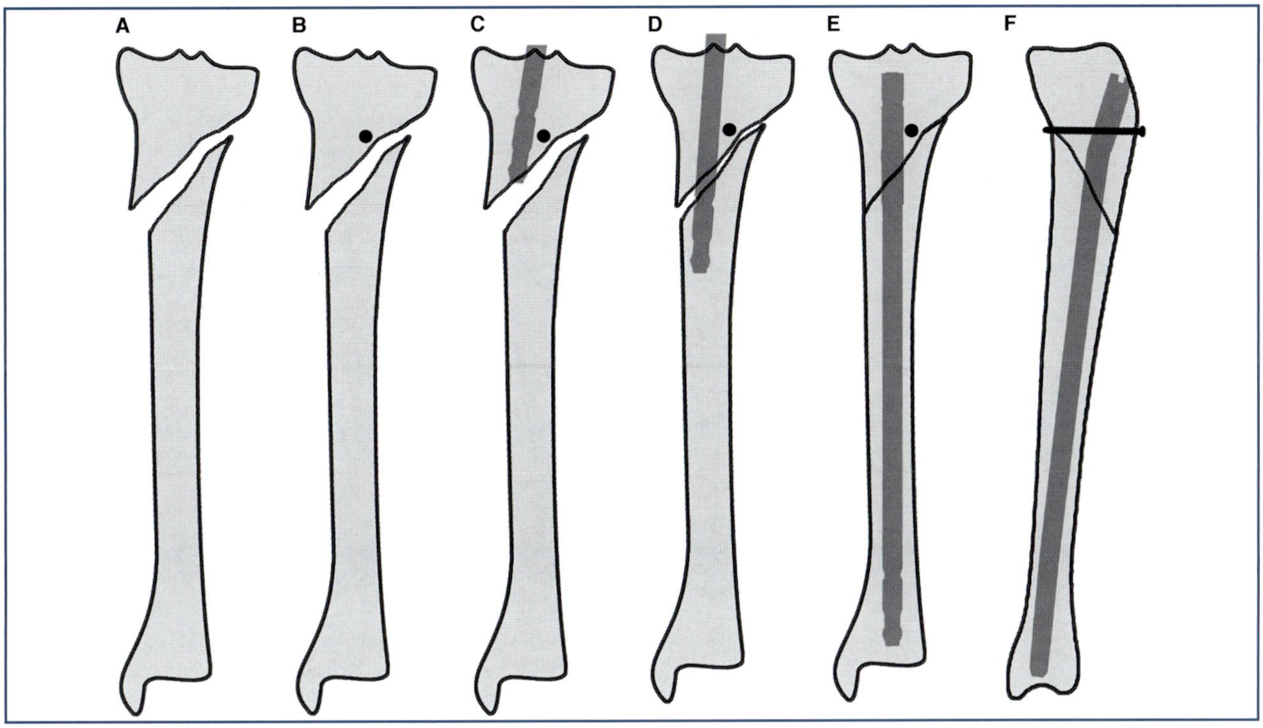

Figure 5 A lateral blocking screw helps prevent valgus angulation. **A,** AP view of a short oblique proximal third tibia fracture. **B,** A blocking screw is placed just lateral to the central axis in an anterior to posterior direction. **C,** The nail is passed medial to the blocking screw. **D,** The valgus angulation begins to be corrected as the nail is passed across the fracture site. **E,** The fracture is properly reduced after the nail is inserted completely. **F,** Lateral view of the tibia following insertion of the nail and blocking screw.

most tibial shaft fractures, minimally invasive percutaneous plating is evolving as a rational treatment alternative for complex tibial shaft fractures, especially those with intra-articular extension.[11] With percutaneous plating there is less disruption of the extraosseous blood supply and the local tissues; both are considered advantages and thought to be critical in preventing the soft-tissue complications and delayed healing often associated with open plating methods for the tibia.[12-14] In their study of 21 distal tibia fractures treated with percutaneous plating, Oh and associates[14] recently reported that all fractures healed after the index procedure without malalignment and without infectious or soft-tissue complications. Collinge and associates[11] reported in 2000 that 17 patients with tibial shaft fractures and associated severe soft-tissue injuries were treated successfully with percutaneous plating. Osteomyelitis developed in only one patient; none had malalignment.

Case Management and Outcome Summary

Two days after the original injury, the patient returned to surgery for revision IM nailing to include the use of blocking screws. If satisfactory alignment could not be obtained with this approach, a secondary plan called for removal of the IM nail and definitive treatment in an external fixator, or possibly open reduction and internal fixation with plates and screws, depending on the condition of the soft-tissue envelope. Scrutinizing the initial and postoperative radiographs was critical to selecting an appropriate operative strategy for correcting the valgus malalignment. The entry point used for the original nail was appropriate, which was fortunate because revising the starting point for an IM nail can be difficult because the nail tends to preferentially enter the previous entry hole.

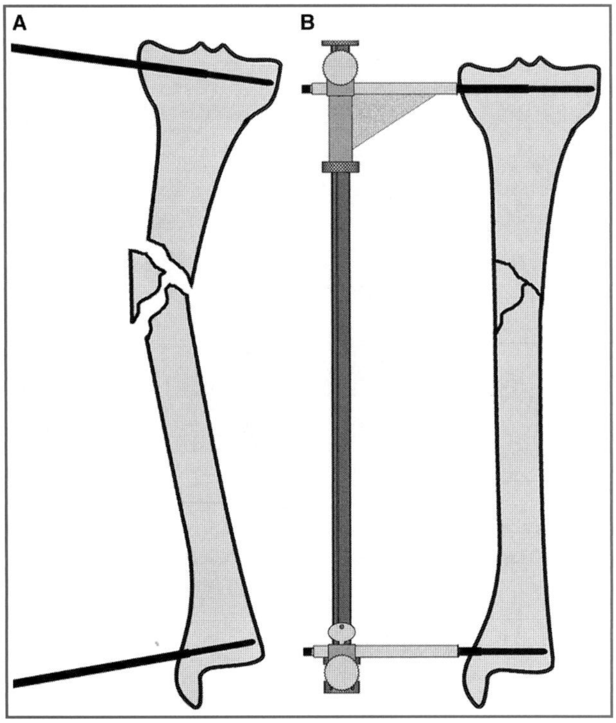

Figure 6 Use of a femoral distractor to help correct coronal plane malalignment. **A,** Pins are placed parallel to the knee and ankle joints. **B,** Alignment is corrected after the femoral distractor is applied.

The principal problem in this case was that the nail failed to be properly aligned within the proximal fragment. To correct the valgus deformity, the nail would need to follow a new path, colinear with the long axis of the proximal fragment. The preoperative plan called for placing blocking screws in the distal portion of the proximal fragment. The most important blocking screw in this case would be the lateral blocking screw. This screw should be placed from anterior to posterior in the distal portion of the proximal fragment, slightly lateral to the long axis. The IM nail would be inserted through the original starting point and medial to this blocking screw, forcing proper alignment in the proximal fragment in the coronal plane. The preoperative plan also called for use of a posterior blocking screw to control the apex anterior angulation that is often associated with proximal tibia fractures. This screw would be placed from medial to lateral in the distal portion of the proximal fracture fragment just posterior to the central axis. Passing the nail anterior to this blocking screw would align the nail in the proximal fragment in the sagittal plane.

In general, the preoperative plan was executed intraoperatively. Through the previous surgical incisions, the interlocking bolts were removed, and the top of the nail was exposed. The extraction device was attached, and the nail completely removed from the tibia. The wound was débrided and then irrigated with pulsatile lavage, including the fracture site. The nail was removed before irrigation and débridement of the open fracture to allow better access to the intramedullary space. Because the wound was generally clean and without significant amounts of nonviable tissue, it was closed definitively.

Next, the blocking screws were placed. This part of the procedure is highly dependent on obtaining satisfactory fluoroscopic images. The hip and knee were extended, and the distal portion of the limb was stabilized by an assistant. A true AP fluoroscopic radiograph centered at the insertion site of the lateral blocking screw confirmed positioning. Through a percutaneous wound, in a fashion similar to freehand interlocking, a 3.5-mm cortical screw was then placed into the distal lateral portion of the proximal fracture fragment and positioned so that when the nail passed medial to the screw, the nail would be centered in the proximal fragment at this level. (I now recommend interlocking bolts rather than 3.5-mm screws because of their increased strength.) The posterior blocking screw was then inserted with the leg elevated to provide an unencumbered lateral fluoroscopic view. Through a percutaneous medial wound, the posterior blocking screw was placed in the distal portion of the proximal fragment, just posterior to long axis. This screw was placed so that when the nail passed anterior to this screw, it would be aligned in the center of the proximal fragment on a lateral radiograph.

Since the previous IM nail was of satisfactory diameter and length, it was reused. Alternatively, a cannulated nail with a flexible guide wire could be used to facilitate insertion past the blocking screws. The nail was assembled to the outrigger, and with the knee flexed approximately 110°, it was introduced into the original entry hole. Using manual forces, the nail was directed medial and anterior to the lateral and posterior blocking screws, respectively. Once the nail had been successfully navigated to the fracture site, the fracture was manually reduced with attention to varus-valgus, anterior-posterior, and rotational align-

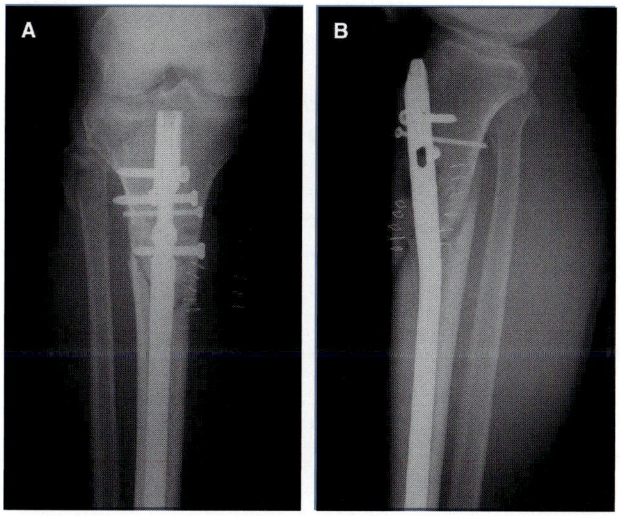

Figure 7 AP (**A**) and lateral (**B**) views after revision IM nailing with blocking screws.

ment. The nail was then inserted to the proper depth into the distal fragment using fluoroscopic guidance. Fracture alignment and nail position were confirmed with AP and lateral radiographs at three locations—the knee, the fracture site, and the distal tip of the nail. These three views were obtained to ensure that parallax would not distort the radiographic findings. The nail was then locked using an outrigger for the proximal interlocking bolts and using a standard freehand method for the distal interlocking bolts (**Figure** 7).

The patient was given intravenous antibiotics for 48 hours because of the open nature of the fracture and then discharged home with instructions for toe-touch weight bearing. Weight-bearing status gradually increased in subsequent weeks until by the sixth week after he was injured, the patient could bear full weight. Serial radiographs revealed that satisfactory alignment and interval healing were achieved. Ten weeks after the injury, he was ambulating with full weight bearing and without assistive devices. He re-

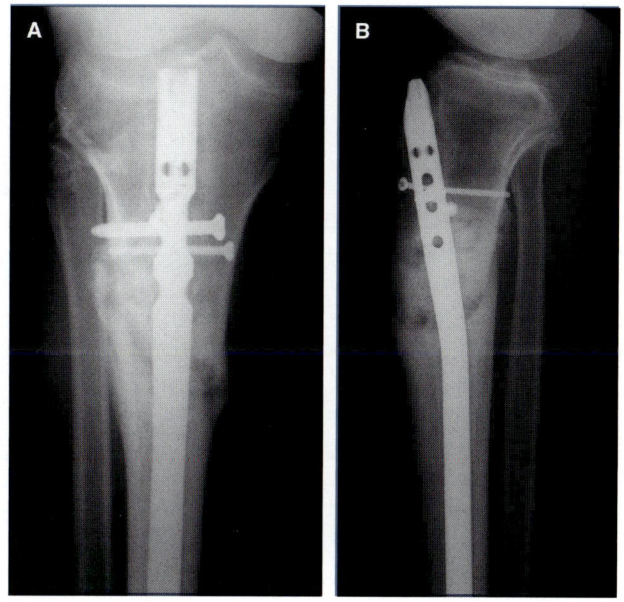

Figure 8 AP (**A**) and lateral (**B**) views obtained 1 year after injury show that satisfactory alignment and interval healing have been achieved.

turned to his job, and at 1 year later had a satisfactory result (**Figure** 8).

Strategies to Minimize Common Complications

In this case, the problems made were technical in nature. When treating end-segment tibia fractures, it is critical to recognize the potential for malalignment. A thorough preoperative plan with contingencies would likely have avoided the problem. I prefer to use blocking screws to avoid malalignment when using IM nailing to treat proximal tibia fractures. Newer minimally invasive plating techniques may prove to be another satisfactory method of treating these fractures.

References

1. Freedman EL, Johnson EE: Radiographic analysis of tibial fracture malalignment following intramedullary nailing. *Clin Orthop* 1995; 25-33.
2. Buehler KC, Green J, Woll TS, Duwelius PJ: A technique for intramedullary nailing of proximal third tibia fractures. *J Orthop Trauma* 1997;11:218-223.
3. Lang GJ, Cohen BE, Bosse MJ, Kellam JF: Proximal third tibial shaft fractures. Should they be nailed? *Clin Orthop* 1995;64-74.
4. Henley MB, Meier M, Tencer AF: Influences of some design parameters on the biomechanics of the unreamed tibial intramedullary

nail. *J Orthop Trauma* 1993; 7:311-319.

5. Ahlers J, von Issendorff WD: Haufigkeit und ursachen von fehlstellungen nach unterschenkelmarknagelungen. *Unfallchirurgie* 1992;18:31-36.
6. Koval KJ, Clapper MF, Brumback RJ, et al: Complications of reamed intramedullary nailing of the tibia. *J Orthop Trauma* 1991;5:184-189.
7. Krettek C, Stephan C, Schandelmaier P, Richter M, Pape HC, Miclau T: The use of Poller screws as blocking screws in stabilising tibial fractures treated with small diameter intramedullary nails. *J Bone Joint Surg Br* 1999;81:963-968.
8. Ricci WM, O'Boyle M, Borrelli J, Bellabarba C, Sanders R: Fractures of the proximal third of the tibial shaft treated with intramedullary nails and blocking screws. *J Orthop Trauma* 2001;15:264-270.
9. Krettek C, Miclau T, Schandelmaier P, Stephan C, Mohlmann U, Tscherne H: The mechanical effect of blocking screws ("Poller screws") in stabilizing tibia fractures with short proximal or distal fragments after insertion of small-diameter intramedullary nails. *J Orthop Trauma* 1999;13:550-553.
10. Tornetta P, Collins E: Semiextended position of intramedullary nailing of the proximal tibia. *Clin Orthop* 1996;185-189.
11. Collinge C, Sanders R, DiPasquale T: Treatment of complex tibial periarticular fractures using percutaneous techniques. *Clin Orthop* 2000;69-77.
12. Borrelli J Jr, Prickett W, Song E, Becker D, Ricci W: Extraosseous blood supply of the tibia and the effects of different plating techniques: A human cadaveric study. *J Orthop Trauma* 2002;16:691-695.
13. Collinge CA, Sanders RW: Percutaneous plating in the lower extremity. *J Am Acad Orthop Surg* 2000;8:211-216.
14. Oh CW, Kyung HS, Park IH, Kim PT, Ihn JC: Distal tibia metaphyseal fractures treated by percutaneous plate osteosynthesis. *Clin Orthop* 2003;286-291.

Chapter 3

Acute Infection After Open Fracture

William M. Ricci, MD

Case Presentation

History

A 41-year-old male pedestrian was struck by a motor vehicle that was traveling approximately 40 miles per hour. Upon arrival at the emergency department, the patient reported right lower extremity pain, and he had an obvious deformity, bleeding, and an open wound. The medical history revealed that he did not have diabetes mellitus and was otherwise healthy with no other history of injury to the affected leg. He reported a 20-year history of smoking 1½ packs of cigarettes per day.

On initial examination, he appeared to be a well-developed, well-nourished man with an acute injury. The right lower extremity had a large open wound about the anterior medial pretibial region, with bone protruding at 90° to the long axis (**Figure 1**). Pulses were slightly diminished on the right side, sensation was intact to light touch, and distal motor function was intact. The left leg was normal on physical examination. No other injuries or abnormalities were noted on physical examination.

AP and lateral radiographs showed segmental tibia and fibula fractures, with comminution of the proximal fracture site located in the proximal one third of the tibial shaft (**Figure 2**). The distal fracture site was located at the junction of the middle and distal thirds of the tibia and was also comminuted. The segmental fracture fragment measured approximately 12 cm in length and was oriented 90° to the long axis, corresponding with the physical examination findings. The fibular fracture was segmental at the same levels as the tibia fracture. Based on his clinical presentation and radiographs, an initial diagnosis of grade IIIB open tibia and fibula fractures was made.

Initial Management

The patient was taken emergently to the operating room for irrigation, débridement, and stabilization. The wound edges were débrided sharply, and all nonviable muscle and soft tissues were débrided as well. Comminuted fracture fragments devoid of soft-tissue attachments at the proximal and distal segmental fracture sites also were removed. The wound was irrigated with 9 L of normal saline solution using a pulsatile irrigation system.

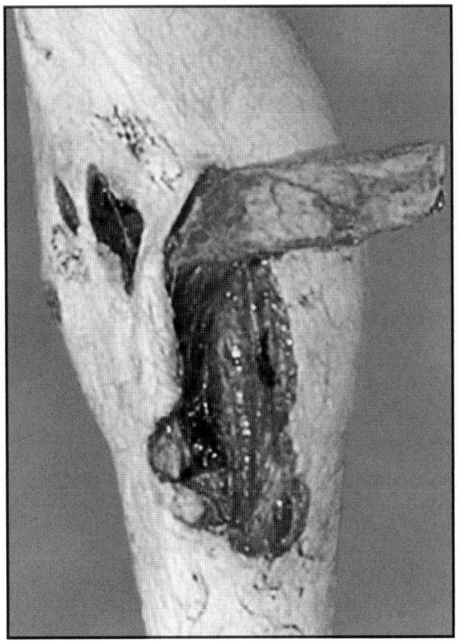

Figure 1 Clinical photograph of the injured extremity.

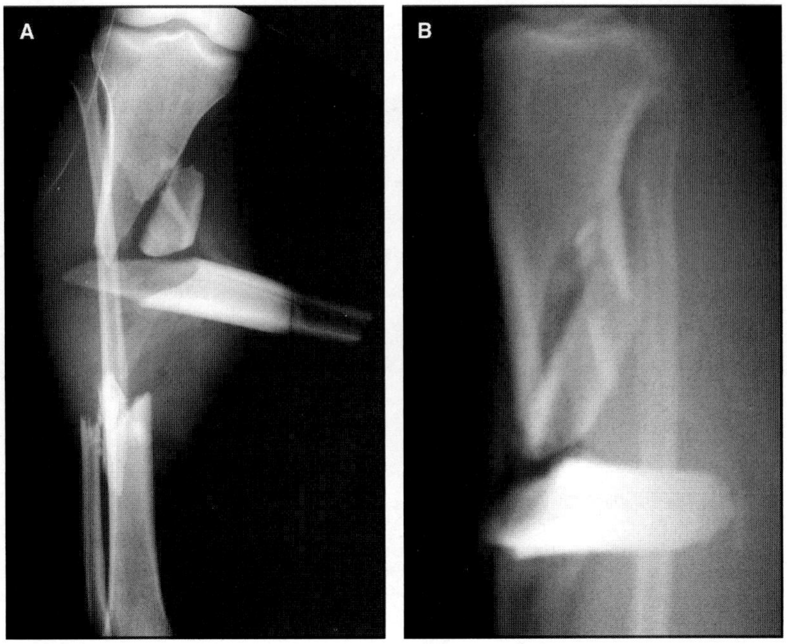

Figure 2 AP (A) and lateral (B) radiographs showing segmental tibia and fibula fractures.

The dilemma in this case was the fate of the large segmental fracture fragment. The distal half of the fragment was clearly stripped of all meaningful soft tissues and blood supply. However, the proximal one third had satisfactory soft-tissue attachments laterally. The decision was made to save the entire fragment.

Stabilization with an intramedullary (IM) nail ensued. Blocking screws were used in the proximal fragment to control angulation at the proximal segmental fracture site. The nail was inserted in a nonreamed fashion to avoid further tearing of the soft-tissue attachments by spinning the segmental fracture fragment and to minimize disruption of the endosteal blood supply (**Figure 3**). The nail was locked proximally and distally in static fashion.

The patient then underwent serial irrigation and débridement procedures. The soft-tissue defect was approximately 15 × 10 cm with approximately 10 cm of exposed subcutaneous tibia (**Figure 4**). A medial gastrocnemius flap was used to provide definitive soft-tissue coverage over the defect, and a split-thickness skin graft was placed over the area. Treatment with intravenous cefazolin and gentamicin was initiated at initial presentation and continued until 48 hours after definitive soft-tissue coverage was achieved. The patient was discharged from the hospital 2 days after flap coverage.

Status of Complication

Two weeks after the injury the flap and skin graft were healing well, but the patient noted increased pain, swelling, erythema, and drainage from the margin of the muscle flap during the second postoperative week. Physical examination at this time revealed a well-healed muscle flap with skin graft. However, there was erythema, swelling, tenderness, and drainage from the margin of the flap anteriorly over the distal segmental fracture level (**Figure 5**). Radiographs showed that the IM nail was in good position, alignment of the limb was satisfactory, and there was early evidence of fracture healing of the proximal segmental fracture. However, there was no radiographic evidence of fracture healing at the distal segmental fracture site.

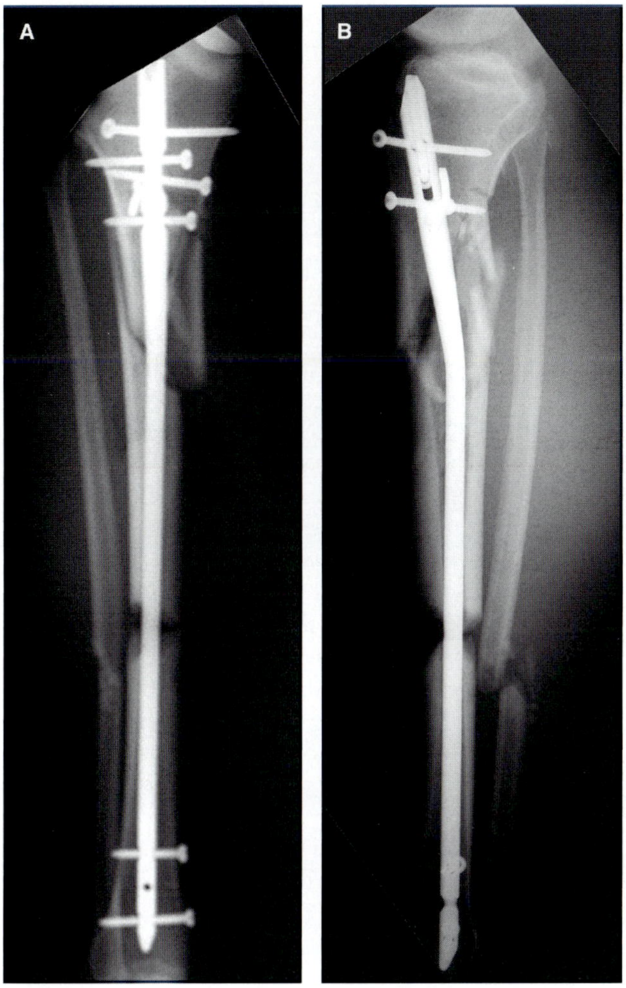

Figure 3 Postoperative AP (**A**) and lateral (**B**) radiographs.

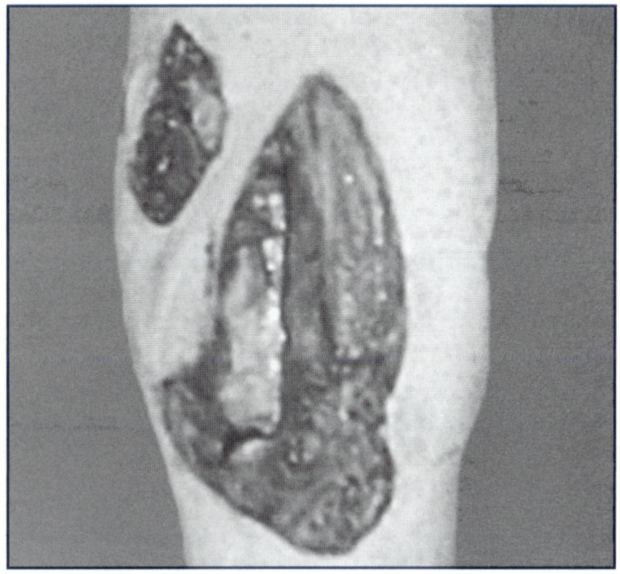

Figure 4 Clinical photograph of soft-tissue defect after serial débridements and IM nailing.

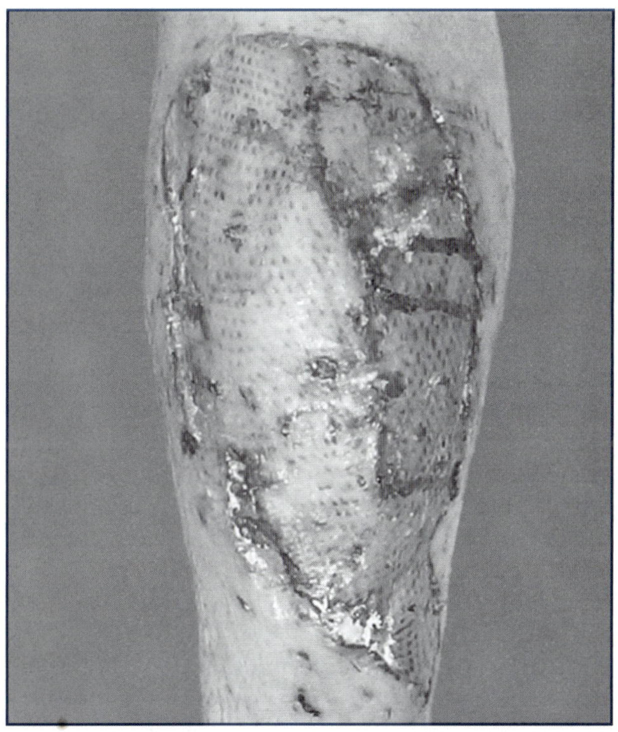

Figure 5 Clinical photograph 3 weeks after injury. Erythema and drainage are present at the margin of the flap, indicative of a deep infection.

DISCUSSION

Recognizing the Problem and Situations at High Risk

Infectious complications are common with open tibia fractures. Recognizing the problem requires following the general principles of identifying infectious complications: increasing pain, swelling, erythema, fever, and purulent drainage are well-known signs of infection. In the absence of obvious signs of infection, the orthopaedist must rely on more indirect markers. Radiographs of open fractures often lack the characteristic periosteal reaction seen with osteomyelitis in other situations. This difference occurs because the regional soft-tissue and periosteal damage that occurs with trauma can inhibit such a hypertrophic reaction. Similarly, in the context of significant local injury, false-negative results can occur on bone scans. Hematologic studies, including white blood cell count with differential, erythrocyte sedimentation rate (ESR), and C-reactive protein (CRP) are useful adjuncts. Elevation of any of these markers can indicate infection. The CRP levels rise more quickly with acute infection and fall more quickly after treatment than the ESR.[1]

This case represents a high-risk situation for infection. A potentially nonviable segment of bone was left in situ in an area of high-energy trauma. When large fragments of bone are deliberately left in situ, the risk of infection is increased given the marginal viability of the bone fragment. In situations of open fracture in which stripped segments of osteoarticular bone are preserved, the risk of infection is unavoidably high. Articular fragments are generally irreplaceable; therefore, they should be preserved whenever possible.

Managing Infection

Management of an acute infection associated with an open fracture first requires removal of all nonviable bone, except for articular fragments that may be salvageable with aggressive sequential irrigation and débridement and administration of local antibiotic. Débridement without a tourniquet can be helpful to evaluate the bleeding potential of the bone. Removal of internal fixation devices in this situation remains controversial. Some authors suggest that a stable fixation device that is performing well should be left in place to promote union; if necessary it can be removed after bone healing. Alternatively, stabilization with external fixation that spans the infected area should be considered. Irrigation and débridement should be performed at least twice (if not more) or until there is no evidence of purulence or further tissue destruction.

Administration of local antibiotics (tailored to the sensitivities of culture results) has been advocated as an adjunct to intravenous antibiotics.[2] A swab sample obtained from the deep tissue and a piece of bone should be sent for initial aerobic and anaerobic cultures. In general, cultures need not be repeated at successive débridements as long as the patient demonstrates a clinical response to the treatment protocol. In immunocompromised patients or those with a history of travel to areas with endemic atypical infections, fungal and tuberculosis cultures are warranted as well.

Multiple local antibiotic delivery systems have been described.[3] Perhaps the most popular delivery system is antibiotic-impregnated polymethylmethacrylate (PMMA) beads. Tobramycin is the most common antibiotic used. This system is considered advantageous because beads offer a high surface area, which delivers high initial local concentrations of antibiotic. The disadvantage of this system is the lack of any structural support and the need for removal, as beads become local foreign bodies without antibiotic potential after approximately 6 weeks.

Antibiotic-impregnated calcium sulfate pellets have been approved and used in Europe. In the United States, calcium sulfate powder can be mixed with antibiotic powder and the appropriate volume of saline solution. Commercially available molds are available to fashion beads. It should be noted that, depending on the antibiotic used, the speed at which polymerization occurs can vary greatly. Manufacturers offer both regular and fast-cure versions. An IM rod made of PMMA impregnated with antibiotic also has been described.[4] This delivery system offers some degree of stabilization and may obviate the need for external fixation.

I recommend removal of local hardware and application of an external fixation frame that spans the zone of infection for initial management of acute infection associated with open tibial fracture. Serial débridements should follow with implantation of antibiotic-impregnated PMMA beads at the site of infection. With definitive closure of the wound, I prefer antibiotic-impregnated calcium sulfate pellets to fill any dead space because union occasionally occurs during the period of IV antibiotic therapy. In these instances, subsequent removal of beads is avoided. The duration of IV antibiotic therapy is usually at least 6 weeks. If the patient has no signs or symptoms of infection and the CRP level has returned to normal or near normal with appropriate trends, any remaining bone void is filled with autologous iliac crest bone graft, which is usually harvested with acetabular reamers.[5] The graft material can be mixed with cal-

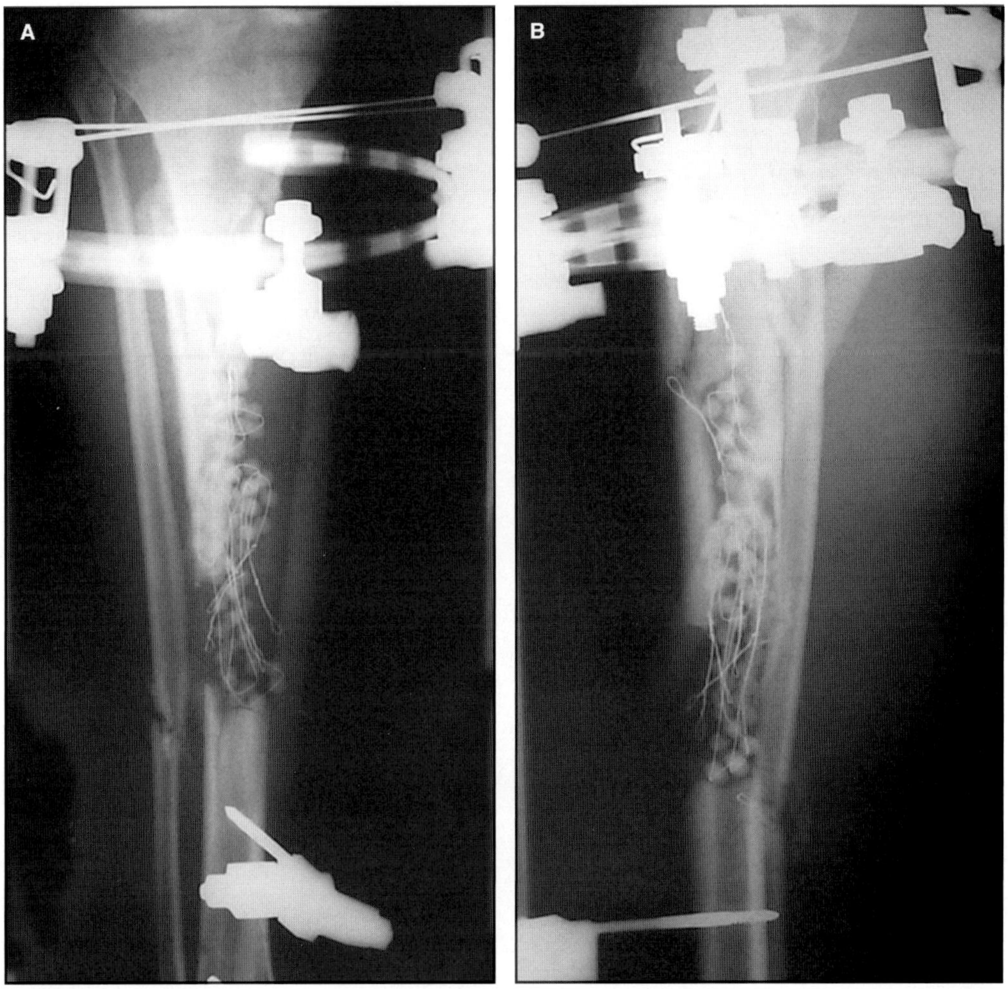

Figure 6 AP (**A**) and lateral (**B**) radiographs after débridement of nonviable bone, application of a hybrid external fixator, and insertion of antibiotic-impregnated PMMA beads in the bone defect.

cium sulfate pellets impregnated with antibiotics to provide both volume expansion and local antibiotic delivery.

Preventing Infection

The most important step in reducing the risk of infection after open tibia fractures is ensuring adequate débridement of nonviable soft and hard tissues. Certainly, any nonarticular free piece of bone, regardless of its size, should be removed. Several authors have reported successful reimplantation of large free structural fragments of femur following sterilization.[6-8] This strategy, however, should be considered an exception for any bone and has not been described for the tibia. Osteoarticular fragments, at times, need to be preserved. In these situations, prolonged antibiotic suppression should be considered as should local delivery of antibiotics in the acute phase.

The approach to treatment that is most appropriate for patients with open tibial shaft fractures, specifically reamed IM nailing, unreamed nailing, or external fixation, has been widely debated and remains controversial. Reaming has proven advantages to promote healing for IM nailing of closed tibia fractures.[9-11] With open fractures in which the periosteal blood supply is damaged from the initial trauma, in-

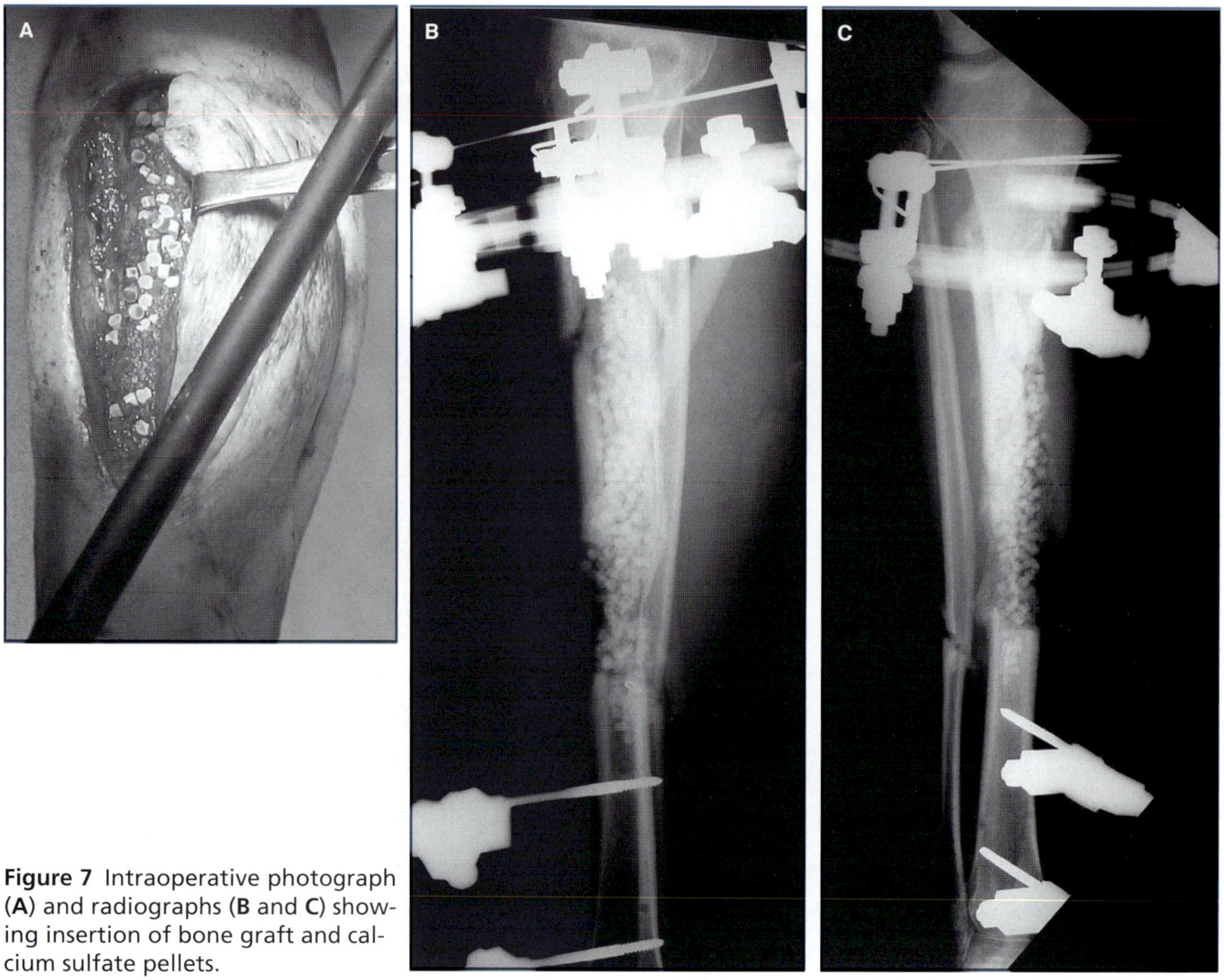

Figure 7 Intraoperative photograph (**A**) and radiographs (**B** and **C**) showing insertion of bone graft and calcium sulfate pellets.

jury to the endosteal blood supply caused by the reaming process is thought to theoretically increase the risk of infection.

Many retrospective[12-18] and several prospective[11,19-21] studies have addressed this issue, but a clear consensus remains illusive. Evidence supporting all three aforementioned treatment modalities can be found. In general, the severity of the soft-tissue injury appears to be the most important factor related to healing and infectious complications.

I believe reaming can be safely used during tibia nailing as long as great care is taken to minimize unnecessary injury to the bone. Specifically, minimal reaming of cortical bone is important, as is use of sharp reamers with a proper flute design to reduce the risks of heat necrosis and subsequent infectious complications.

Case Management and Outcome Summary

In this case, the patient was brought to the operating suite, and the margin of the gastrocnemius flap was opened during surgery over the distal segmental fracture site. The distal one third of the segmental fracture fragment was pearly white and clearly nonviable; approximately 8 cm of the anterior portion of this fragment was débrided with a high-speed burr. The posterior and proximal portions showed good punctate bleeding and were clearly viable; therefore, these fragments were retained in situ. The IM nail and all hardware were removed, and a spanning external fixator was placed across the zone of infection. Two half pins were placed in the distal fragment, and a 5/8 ring and thin wires were placed across the proximal fragment, outside the zone of infection. The patient underwent three consecutive irrigation and débridement procedures. Antibiotic-impregnated PMMA beads were used to provide local antibiotic delivery between débridement procedures (**Figure 6**). Cultures were obtained only at the first irrigation and débridement procedure because the patient responded to treatment. Antibiotic-impregnated calcium sulfate pellets were used to provide local antibiotic coverage after the final irrigation and débridement procedure.

Six weeks after final irrigation and débridement, there were no clinical signs of infection, the patient was afebrile, the wound showed no signs of erythema, drainage, or tenderness. The patient's ESR and CRP normalized. Radiographs showed signs of healing at the proximal segmental fracture site and posterior bridging of bone across the distal site. There was approximately a 10-cm anterior defect.

At 10 weeks, the patient underwent iliac crest bone grafting supplemented with calcium sulfate pellets (**Figure 7**). The external fixator remained in place to provide additional stabilization. Serial radiographs showed gradual incorporation of the bone graft. Subsequently, the patient gradually increased weight bearing in the external fixator frame. Three months after bone grafting, the external fixator frame was removed and a cast applied. His weight-bearing status advanced gradually from toe-touch weight bearing to full weight bearing in a brace over the subsequent 3 months. One year after the initial injury, the bone was solidly healed, and the patient was able to bear full weight without assistive devices and was without any sign of infection (**Figure 8**). Suppressive antibiotic therapy was discontinued.

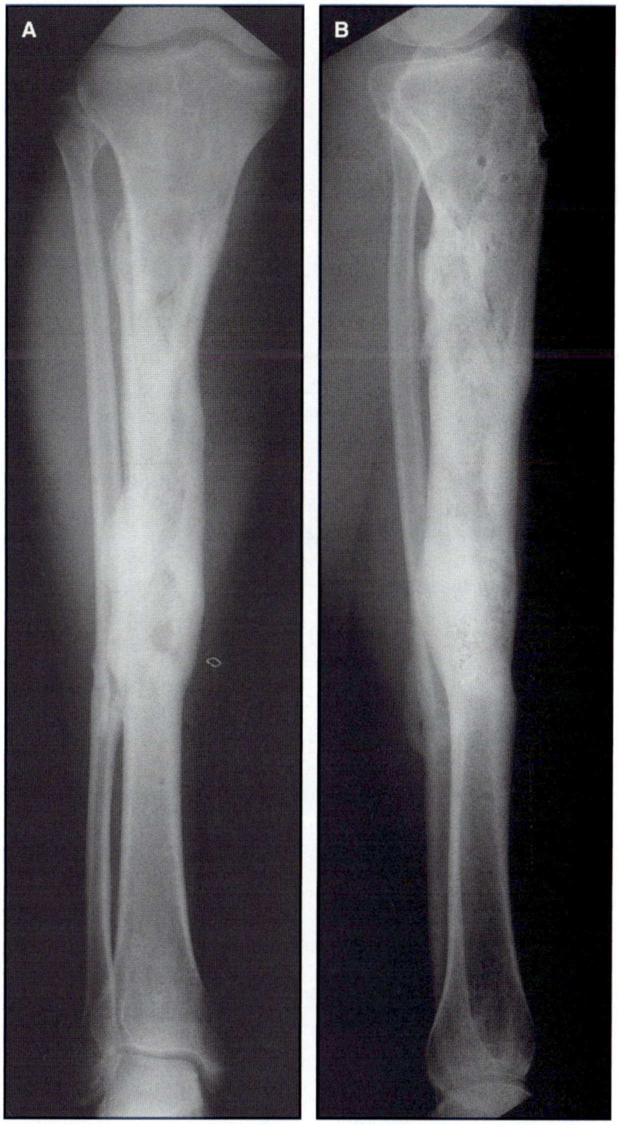

Figure 8 AP (**A**) and lateral (**B**) radiographs 1 year after injury showing fracture healing and consolidation of the bone grafted defect.

Strategies to Minimize Common Complications

In this case, the decision to retain a portion of nonviable bone potentially led to the infectious complication. It is often difficult for the orthopaedic surgeon to discard such large pieces of bone. In this case, because the patient responded so well to the operative débridements and IV antibiotic treatment, there were few long-term sequelae from the infection. In retrospect, the distal portion of the segmental fracture fragment should have been resected at the time of initial trauma. A circular external fixator applied at the time of initial bony stabilization would have minimized the amount of foreign material in the zone of injury and may have further decreased the risk of infection.

References

1. Unkila-Kallio L, Kallio MJ, Eskola J, Peltola H: Serum C-reactive protein, erythrocyte sedimentation rate, and white blood cell count in acute hematogenous osteomyelitis of children. *Pediatrics* 1994;93:59-62.
2. Henry SL, Ostermann PA, Seligson D: The antibiotic bead pouch technique. The management of severe compound fractures. *Clin Orthop* 1993;295:54-62.
3. Holtom PD, Patzakis MJ: Newer methods of antimicrobial delivery for bone and joint infections. *Instr Course Lect* 2003;52:745-749.
4. Paley D, Herzenberg JE: Intramedullary infections treated with antibiotic cement rods: Preliminary results in nine cases. *J Orthop Trauma* 2002;16:723-729.
5. Westrich GH, Geller DS, O'Malley MJ, Deland JT, Helfet DL: Anterior iliac crest bone graft harvesting using the corticocancellous reamer system. *J Orthop Trauma* 2001;15:500-506.
6. Kao JT, Comstock C: Reimplantation of a contaminated and devitalized bone fragment after autoclaving in an open fracture. *J Orthop Trauma* 1995;9:336-340.
7. Mazurek MT, Pennington SE, Mills WJ: Successful reimplantation of a large segment of femoral shaft in a type IIIA open femur fracture: A case report. *J Orthop Trauma* 2003;17:295-299.
8. Moosazadeh K: Successful reimplantation of retrieved large segment of open femoral fracture: Case report. *J Trauma* 2002;53:133-138.
9. Bhandari M: Guyatt GH, Tong D, Adili A, Shaughnessy SG: Reamed versus nonreamed intramedullary nailing of lower extremity long bone fractures: A systematic overview and meta-analysis. *J Orthop Trauma* 2000;14:2-9.
10. Court-Brown CM, Will E, Christie J, McQueen MM: Reamed or unreamed nailing for closed tibial fractures. A prospective study in Tscherne C1 fractures. *J Bone Joint Surg Br* 1996;78:580-583.
11. Finkemeier CG, Schmidt AH, Kyle RF, Templeman DC, Varecka TF: A prospective, randomized study of intramedullary nails inserted with and without reaming for the treatment of open and closed fractures of the tibial shaft. *J Orthop Trauma* 2000;14:187-193.
12. Court-Brown CM, McQueen MM, Quaba AA, Christie J: Locked intramedullary nailing of open tibial fractures. *J Bone Joint Surg Br* 1991;73:959-964.
13. Dickson KF, Hoffman WY, Delgado ED, Contreras DM: Unreamed rod with early wound closure for grade IIIA and IIIB open tibial fractures: Analysis of 40 consecutive patients. *Orthopedics* 1998;21:531-535.
14. Keating JF, O'Brien PI, Blachut PA, Meek RN, Broekhuyse HM: Reamed interlocking intramedullary nailing of open fractures of the tibia. *Clin Orthop* 1997;338:182-191.
15. Schandelmaier P, Krettek C, Rudolf J, Kohl A, Katz BE, Tscherne H: Superior results of tibial rodding versus external fixation in grade 3B fractures. *Clin Orthop* 1997;342:164-172.
16. Schandelmaier P, Krettek C, Rudolf J, Tscherne H: Outcome of tibial shaft fractures with severe soft tissue injury treated by unreamed nailing versus external fixation. *J Trauma* 1995;39:707-711.
17. Shannon FJ, Mullett H, O'Rourke K: Unreamed intramedullary nail versus external fixation in grade III open tibial fractures. *J Trauma* 2002;52:650-654.
18. Whittle AP, Russell TA, Taylor JC, Lavelle DG: Treatment of open fractures of the tibial shaft with the use of interlocking nailing without reaming. *J Bone Joint Surg Am* 1992;74:1162-1171.
19. Henley MB, Chapman JR, Agel J, Harvey EJ, Whorton AM, Swiontkowski MF: Treatment of type II, IIIA, and IIIB open fractures of the tibial shaft: A prospective comparison of unreamed interlocking intramedullary nails and half-pin external fixators. *J Orthop Trauma* 1998;12:1-7.
20. Tornetta P III, Bergman M, Watnik N, Berkowitz G, Steuer J: Treatment of grade-IIIb open tibial fractures. A prospective randomised comparison of external fixation and non-reamed locked nailing. *J Bone Joint Surg Br* 1994;76:13-19.
21. Tu YK, Lin CH, Su JI, Hsu DT, Chen RJ: Unreamed interlocking nail versus external fixator for open type III tibia fractures. *J Trauma* 1995;39:361-367.

Chapter 4

Aseptic Nonunion after IM Nailing

William M. Ricci, MD

Case Presentation

History

A 68-year-old woman with rheumatoid arthritis and type I diabetes mellitus reported increasing pain in the pretibial region over a period of several weeks without antecedent trauma. She did not smoke and had a history of bilateral total knee arthroplasty. Initial radiographs revealed a transverse nondisplaced stress fracture in the midshaft of the tibia (**Figure 1**). No fibula fracture was seen. The knee prostheses showed no signs of loosening.

Initial Management

The patient was treated with unlocked nonreamed intramedullary (IM) nailing of the tibia.

Status of the Complication

Initially, the patient reported partial symptom relief, and weight bearing was allowed to progressively increase as tolerated. After several weeks, she reported increasing pain. Radiographs obtained at this time revealed migration of the IM nail, deformity at the fracture site, and evidence of nonunion (**Figure 2**).

Discussion

Recognizing the Problem and Situations at High Risk

The first step in avoiding nonunion of tibial shaft fractures is to recognize the etiologic factors implicated in aseptic nonunion. These factors fall under four categories: (1) host characteristics (smoking, diabetes mellitus, nutritional status, immunocompetence); (2) fracture characteristics (comminution, fracture pattern, location, bone loss, associated fibula fracture); (3) soft-tissue injury (degree of local soft-tissue injury); and (4) fixation characteristics (degree of stability, degree of additional soft-tissue compromise, alignment, quality of postoperative care).

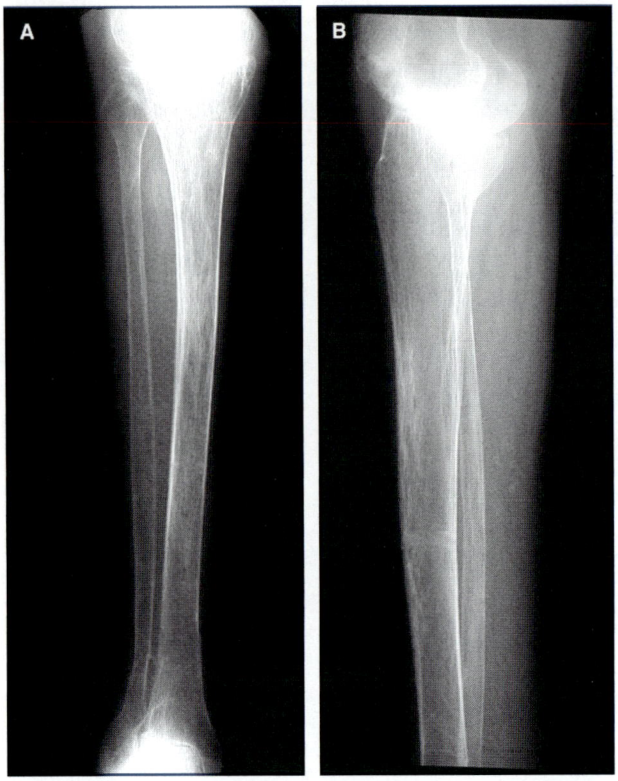

Figure 1 Initial AP (**A**) and lateral (**B**) radiographs showing a nondisplaced midshaft tibial stress fracture.

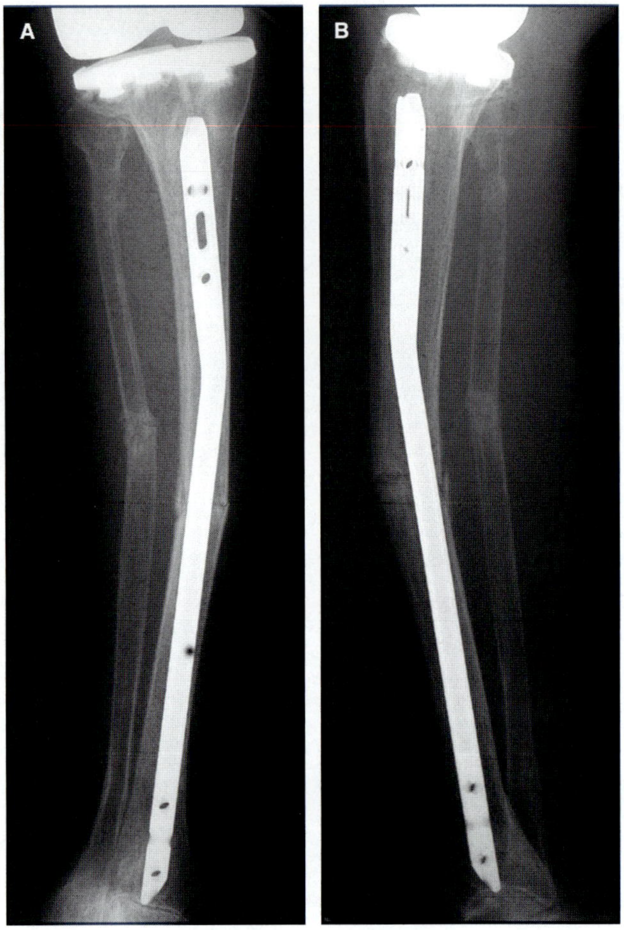

Figure 2 AP (**A**) and lateral (**B**) radiographs showing migration of the nail and deformity at the fracture site. Note the lateral nail profile on the AP view of the tibia.

Host Characteristics

Diabetes mellitus is thought to contribute to delayed healing and higher rates of complications in patients with lower extremity fractures. This association has been clearly shown with ankle fractures. The evidence linking diabetes and delayed healing of tibia fractures, however, is quite limited. In one study,[1] four of six patients with diabetes mellitus experienced nonunion of a tibia fracture. Animal studies report that control of hyperglycemia may improve healing; therefore, patients with diabetes mellitus should be encouraged to strictly control their blood glucose levels, and they should be monitored closely for complications related to fracture healing, infection, and wound complications.

The effect of nonsteroidal anti-inflammatory drugs (NSAIDs) on fracture healing remains controversial. In animal models, nonspecific NSAIDs and, to a lesser degree, COX-2 selective inhibitors have been shown to inhibit fracture healing.[2] Clinically, NSAIDs have been associated with delayed healing and nonunion in patients with femoral shaft fractures.[3] These reports suggest that NSAIDs should be avoided in patients with acute fractures. Précis knowledge of what time period after fracture is most affected by NSAIDs and whether the effect is reversible has yet to be determined. Smoking has also been implicated in both delayed wound and fracture healing.[4] Patients with tibia fractures should be encouraged to stop or at least reduce the number of cigarettes they smoke, especially patients with or at high risk for delayed or nonunion.

Fracture Characteristics/ Soft-tissue Injury

Transverse fracture (relative risk of 20.0) and open fracture (relative risk of 4.32) patterns are associated with revision after tibial shaft fracture.[5] Patients with open fractures and those who sustain high-energy trauma have a higher relative risk for nonunion than those with closed fractures or low-energy trauma, respectively.[6]

Fixation Characteristics

Multiple investigators have reported that reamed IM nailing for closed tibial shaft fractures provides faster and more reliable healing with fewer secondary procedures than unreamed nailing.[7-9] Lack of cortical continuity between fracture ends following fixation has recently been shown to predict the need for revision (relative risk 8.33).[5]

Diagnosis of Nonunion

Nonunion of tibia shaft fractures can be difficult to recognize. In patients who lack bridging bone across a fracture site and report pain on weight bearing, the diagnosis is relatively straightforward. However, accurately identifying bridging callus can be difficult. The reported number of cortices required to confirm radiographic union varies from two cortices on orthogonal views to all four cortices. In addition, the obliquity of a fracture site can obscure accurate identification or absence of bridging callus. There is no gold standard to confirm radiographic union. Advanced imaging studies such as tomography, CT, bone scan, and ultrasound have been used with varying degrees of success.[10]

To further complicate the ability to confirm delayed healing, the definition of delayed and nonunion lacks standardization.[1] Definitions of nonunion range widely from lack of union within a specific time frame (range, 2 months to 1 year),[1,6,11,12] to lack of progressive fracture healing over a 3-month period, to two times the expected healing time of 16 weeks.[1] The time from injury to the diagnosis of delayed union ranges from 1 to 8 months.[11] Given the discrepancy among these definitions, any patient with pain at the fracture site associated with weight bearing and equivocal radiographic evidence of healing should be evaluated for fracture nonunion.

Nonunions can also be characterized by the host response. Hypertrophic nonunions are well vascularized and have abundant callus but usually have poor mechanical stability. Adequate mechanical stability is of paramount importance in treating these nonunions. Atrophic nonunions, in contrast, have poor vascularity and absent callus, and their treatment usually requires biologic stimulation in addition to adequate stability.

Managing Nonunion

The proper timing for surgical intervention for tibial nonunion remains unclear. Surgical intervention is indicated when there is little potential for union without additional treatment. The decision to perform surgery often can be made 3 to 5 months after injury in the absence of progressive signs of fracture healing, but this decision can be delayed if there is evidence of progressive healing.[8,13,14] Treatment method for nonunion depends on multiple factors, including the local biologic response to the fracture (ie, the type of nonunion), the time frame, the previous treatment, and patient comorbidities.

Nonsurgical Treatment

Weight bearing in a cast or brace, following a period in which the patient could not bear weight, can sometimes stimulate progressive fracture consolidation. Functional bracing, usually preceded by fibular ostectomy, has been shown to result in fracture union at a median of 4 months with an average of 5 mm of shortening in 91% of patients.[15] Management of fracture nonunion with external electrical and ultrasound stimulation remains controversial. Compliant patients with aseptic hypertrophic fracture nonunions and no deformity may benefit from these methods. However, noncompliant patients who have deformity or atrophic nonunion have little to gain from these modalities.

Dynamization

Conversion of a static tibial nail to a dynamic construct by removing the interlocking bolts, dynamization, can be used to help promote union in fractures that show poor initial healing response, in delayed unions, and in nonunions. The précis timing of intervention remains unclear because as Wu and Shih reported,[16] the interval from initial nailing to dynamization did not correlate with successful healing; the longest interval from dynamization to successful healing was 20 months. In this study, fracture union was achieved in approximately 50% of patients, with dynamization performed at an average of 7.8 months. Dynamization has been reported to stimulate union in 14% of closed fractures treated with IM nailing at an average of 19 weeks after initial surgery.[6]

Exchange Nailing

Exchange IM nailing of the tibia has proved to be successful in treating nonunion of previously nailed tibia fractures. At an average of 36 weeks from initial treatment, exchange nailing resulted in union in 84% of patients (average, 20 weeks following exchange nailing).[17] Reamed nailing has been successful to treat tibial nonunion, regardless of the initial type of treatment.[18]

Plate Osteosyntheses

Plate osteosyntheses is also very effective in the treatment of tibial nonunion. This technique can be applied to fracture sites along the entire length of the tibia and is especially useful in patients with associated malalignment that requires correction. Adjuvant autologous bone grafting is often used.

This technique is preferred as long as the patient can tolerate its disadvantages, specifically prolonged protected weight bearing and an increased risk of soft-tissue complications. In patients with a compromised soft-tissue envelope surrounding a nonunion site, plate osteosyntheses should be used with extreme caution. Plate fixation without bone grafting is indicated for hypertrophic nonunions in which the local environment requires enhanced fracture stabilization but has viable biology to allow fracture healing.

External Fixation

Small wire circular external fixation is especially useful in treatment of periarticular nonunions. It is also particularly useful in correcting deformities with associated compromise of the soft-tissue envelope. External fixation techniques have a high rate of complications, most commonly relatively minor pin tract problems; they also are technically demanding, have a long and steep learning curve, and often require additional training. The success of external fixation also depends on proper patient selection. Patients must be willing to tolerate close follow-up, the potential for multiple revision surgeries, and the demands of pin care. They also must be psychologically and emotionally capable of enduring months, and sometimes more than a year, of wearing an external fixator.

Bone Grafting

Morcellized autologous cancellous bone graft is considered the standard for promoting healing of an atrophic nonunion and for filling bone voids of up to 6 cm. Posterolateral bone grafting has been advocated for use in nonunions of the middle and distal thirds of the tibia. Such bone grafting technique avoids any skin or soft-tissue deficiencies about the subcutaneous region of the tibia anteromedially. Alternatively, bone grafting through the site of a tibial nonunion can be accomplished when the fracture site is directly exposed for plate fixation. Myriad bone graft substitutes are now available. However, when used for nonunions, only those substitutes that have osteoinductive properties have any role. Substitutes with osteoconductive properties can be useful to expand the volume of an autologous bone graft or to fill metaphyseal bone voids in the acute setting, but these substitutes alone have little role in treatment of tibial nonunions. Percutaneous injection of bone marrow aspirated from the iliac crest has also been advocated in the treatment of tibial nonunions. For this technique to be successful, the marrow must be inserted precisely at the site of nonunion or delayed union, usually under fluoroscopic control. Also, adequate fracture stabilization is necessary for this technique to be successful.

Preventing Nonunion After IM Nailing

Fracture characteristics, soft-tissue injury, and host characteristics are potentially prognostic for nonunion, but surgeons have little control over these factors. Therefore, proper surgical technique is the prin-

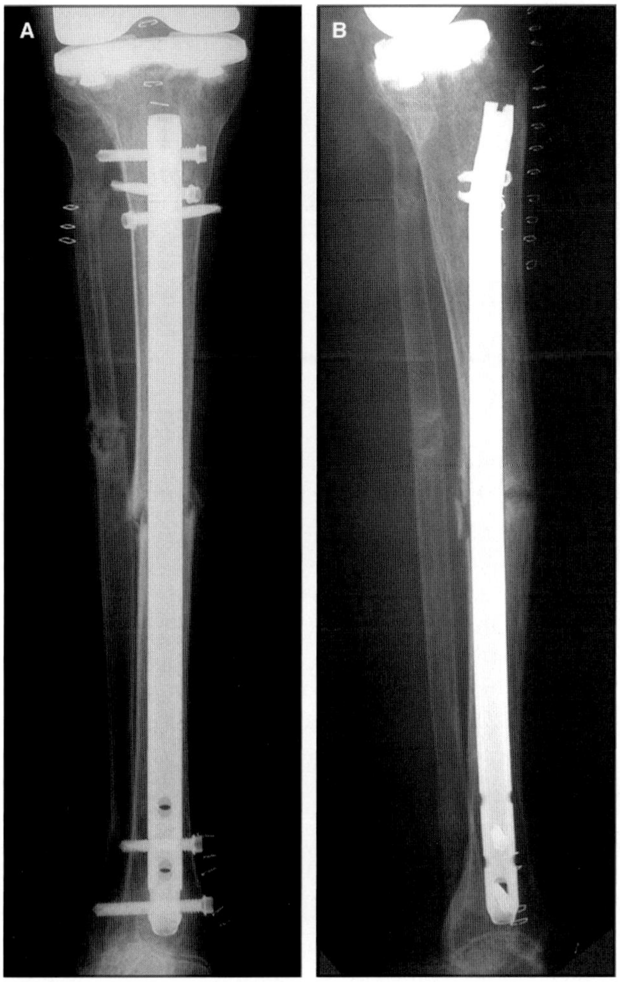

Figure 3 AP (**A**) and lateral (**B**) radiographs after exchange nailing.

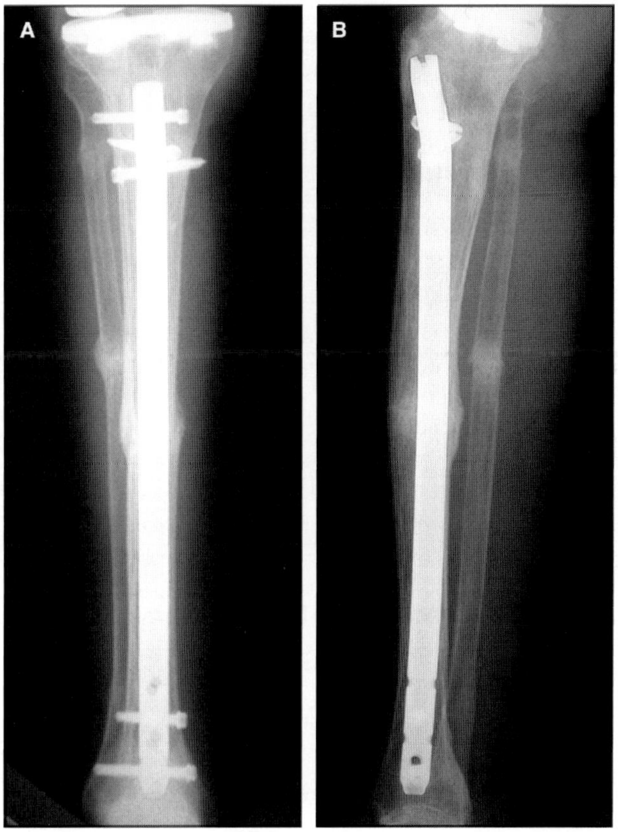

Figure 4 AP (**A**) and lateral (**B**) radiographs obtained 8 months after exchange nailing show the healed fracture.

cipal way in which the surgeon can reduce the risk of nonunion.

Historically, reaming was necessary to enlarge the medullary cavity so that a large-diameter nail, required for adequate strength given the relatively poor mechanical properties of early nails, could be inserted. Reaming also increases the contact area between the endosteal cortical bone and the nail, providing more stability. Aggressive reaming of cortical bone is now believed to be unnecessary.

Proper reaming technique requires that the fracture be reduced during passage of reamers. If not, eccentric reaming will occur, and malalignment may occur when the nail passes through the tract created by the reaming. This problem is especially common in more comminuted fracture patterns. Proper reaming technique also requires using sharp reamers (to minimize generation of thermal necrosis), passing the reamers relatively slowly, and ensuring minimal reaming of endosteal cortical bone (MA Karunakar, et al, Toronto, Canada, unpublished data presented at the Orthopaedic Trauma Association Annual Meeting, 2002). For the tibia, overreaming by 0.5 to 1.5 mm is generally acceptable. Despite laboratory investigations indicating that reaming destroys endosteal circulation and has potentially adverse effects on fracture healing, clinical studies have clearly demonstrated that reaming is advantageous.[8]

Cortical contact at the fracture site should be achieved, especially for transverse fractures. After placement of the nail and proximal interlocking, the insertion handles should be gently tapped with the patient's foot firmly planted on the operating table to reduce fracture gaps. Once satisfactory cortical contact is confirmed on fluoroscopic views, the outrigger can be removed, the knee extended, and distal freehand interlocks placed. Alternatively, some surgeons prefer to insert distal interlocks first, "back slap" the insertion device to compress the fracture site, and then place the proximal interlocking bolts. The method chosen depends, in part, on the individual nail system used, with particular attention to the location and use of dynamic interlocking bolts. These techniques should be used only when a static interlocking bolt is in place. The back slap method may be less advantageous if the nailing system does not allow extension of the knee for distal interlocking with the insertion handle attached.

Case Management and Outcome Summary

Several problems related to the surgical technique were evident in this case. First, the IM nail did not provide any rotational control due to the lack of interlocking bolts. Second, the nail was inserted in a nonreamed fashion. To correct the nonunion, the surgeon decided to remove the initial nail with a plan for exchange nailing. The patient was brought to the operating room, and the old nail was removed through the previous surgical site. A guide wire was then placed down the canal. Reaming was performed at 0.5-mm increments with the tourniquet released until chatter was encountered. A nail that was 1.0 mm in diameter smaller than the final reamer was inserted and then locked at both the proximal and distal ends to control rotational alignment (**Figure 3**). The patient was allowed progressive weight bearing and healed without further complication at 10 weeks after exchange nailing (**Figure 4**).

Strategies to Minimize Common Complications

The decision to treat this patient's stress fracture with an IM nail was a reasonable one. The advantage of IM nailing, especially in elderly or debilitated patients, is the ability to initiate weight bearing earlier. These patients often find it very difficult, or even impossible, to comply with the non–weight-bearing status advocated with nonsurgical treatment of these stress fractures. The two problems in this situation were (1) the lack of IM reaming and (2) the lack of proper interlocking. As previously stated, IM reaming has been associated with higher rates of and faster times to union. Proximal and distal interlocking is necessary to achieve rotational stability. Most modern nailing systems allow such interlocking with the ability for fracture compression through weight bearing via insertion of dynamic interlocking bolts. Following standard modern IM techniques would likely have avoided the complication in this case.

References

1. Loder RT: The influence of diabetes mellitus on the healing of closed fractures. *Clin Orthop* 1988;232:210-216.
2. Gerstenfeld LC, Thiede M, Seibert K, et al: Differential inhibition of fracture healing by non-selective and cyclooxygenase-2 selective non-steroidal anti-inflammatory drugs. *J Orthop Res* 2003;21:670-675.
3. Giannoudis PV, MacDonald DA, Matthews SJ, Smith RM, Furlong AJ, De Boer P: Nonunion of the femoral diaphysis. The influence of reaming and non-steroidal anti-inflammatory drugs. *J Bone Joint Surg Br* 2000;82:655-658.
4. Schmitz MA, Finnegan M, Natarajan R, Champine J: Effect of smoking on tibial shaft fracture healing. *Clin Orthop* 1999;365:184-200.
5. Bhandari M, Tornetta P III, Sprague S, et al: Predictors of reoperation following operative management of fractures of the tibial shaft. *J Orthop Trauma* 2003;17:353-361.
6. Karladani AH, Granhed H, Karrholm J, Styf J: The influence of fracture etiology and type on fracture healing: A review of 104 consecutive tibial shaft fractures. *Arch Orthop Trauma Surg* 2001;121:325-328.
7. Bhandari M, Guyatt GH, Tong D, Adili A, Shaughnessy SG: Reamed versus nonreamed intramedullary nailing of lower extremity long

bone fractures: A systematic overview and meta-analysis. *J Orthop Trauma* 2000;14:2-9.

8. Court-Brown CM, Will E, Christie J, McQueen MM: Reamed or unreamed nailing for closed tibial fractures. A prospective study in Tscherne C1 fractures. *J Bone Joint Surg Br* 1996;78:580-583.
9. Finkemeier CG, Schmidt AH, Kyle RF, Templeman DC, Varecka TF: A prospective, randomized study of intramedullary nails inserted with and without reaming for the treatment of open and closed fractures of the tibial shaft. *J Orthop Trauma* 2000;14:187-193.
10. Moed BR, et al: Ultrasound for the early diagnosis of tibial fracture healing after static interlocked nailing without reaming: Clinical results. *J Orthop Trauma* 1998;12: 206-213.
11. Bhandari M, Guyatt GH, Swiontkowski MF, Tornetta P III, Sprague S, Schemitsch EH: A lack of consensus in the assessment of fracture healing among orthopaedic surgeons. *J Orthop Trauma* 2002;16: 562-566.
12. Bone LB, Sucato D, Stegemann PM, Rohrbacher BJ: Displaced isolated fractures of the tibial shaft treated with either a cast or intramedullary nailing. An outcome analysis of matched pairs of patients. *J Bone Joint Surg Am* 1997; 79:1336-1341.
13. Fischer MD, Gustilo RB, Varecka TF: The timing of flap coverage, bone-grafting, and intramedullary nailing in patients who have a fracture of the tibial shaft with extensive soft-tissue injury. *J Bone Joint Surg Am* 1991;73:1316-1322.
14. Gustilo RB, Mendoza RM, Williams DN: Problems in the management of type III (severe) open fractures: A new classification of type III open fractures. *J Trauma* 1984;24:742-746.
15. Sarmiento A, Burkhalter WE, Latta LL: Functional bracing in the treatment of delayed union and nonunion of the tibia. *Int Orthop* 2003;27:26-29.
16. Wu CC, Shih CH: Effect of dynamization of a static interlocking nail on fracture healing. *Can J Surg* 1993;36:302-306.
17. Mercado EM, Lim EV, Stern PJ, Aquino NJ: Exchange nailing for failure of initially rodded tibial shaft fractures. *Orthopedics* 2001; 24:757-762.
18. Megas P, Panagiotopoulos E, Skriviliotakis S, Lambiris E: Intramedullary nailing in the treatment of aseptic tibial nonunion. *Injury* 2001;32:233-239.

Chapter 5

Failure of Nonunion Repair

Joseph Borrelli, Jr, MD

Case Presentation

History

A 39-year-old woman sustained a closed oblique fracture of the midshaft of her right tibia and fibula in a fall from a 3-foot ladder (**Figure 1**). Initial assessment revealed that the patient was generally healthy, did not smoke or have diabetes mellitus, and had an isolated, minimally displaced fracture of the tibial shaft.

Initial Management

Nonsurgical management was initiated because of the nature of the fracture. A long leg cast was applied, and the patient was limited to toe-touch weight bearing with the use of crutches. After 6 weeks, radiographs revealed progressive healing and no change in fracture alignment. The cast was converted to a patellar tendon-bearing cast, and weight bearing was advanced. After 4 additional weeks, the cast was removed, a prefabricated fracture brace was applied, and she was advanced to full weight bearing. Pain at the fracture site with weight bearing persisted, and serial radiographs obtained from this point on showed a fracture nonunion. Autologous bone marrow aspirate from the iliac crest was injected into the nonunion site to stimulate fracture healing.[1] Despite this treatment, nonunion and pain persisted. Three years after the injury, she was referred for definitive treatment of the nonunion.

Status of the Complication

Upon presentation, the patient had an obvious deformity of the right tibia with gross motion and pain at the nonunion site with varus and valgus stressing. There were no signs or symptoms of infection, and the limb was neurovascularly intact. Radiographs revealed an oligotrophic nonunion despite two attempts at nonunion repair with autologous bone marrow aspiration and injection (**Figure 2**).

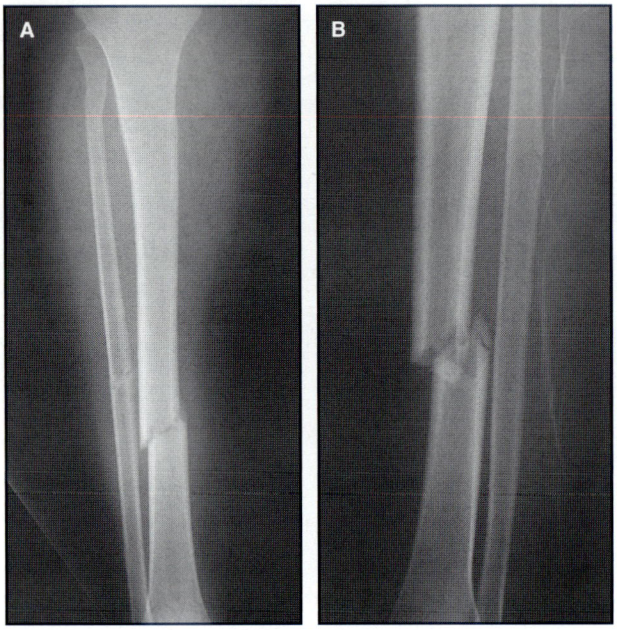

Figure 1 Initial AP (**A**) and lateral (**B**) radiographs demonstrating midshaft fractures of the tibia and fibula.

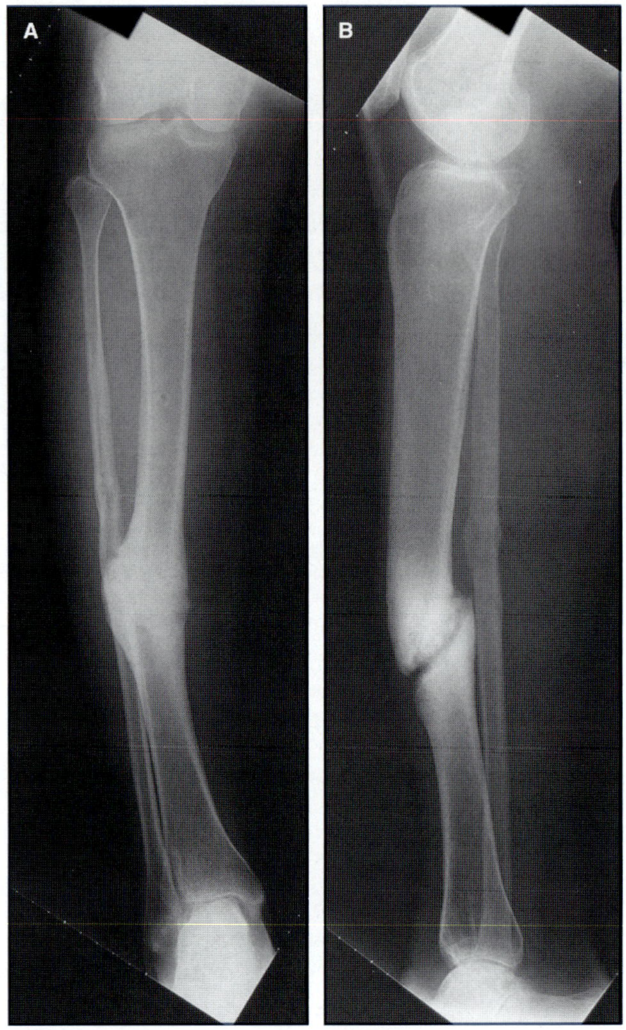

Figure 2 AP (**A**) and lateral (**B**) radiographs demonstrating a midshaft tibial oligotrophic nonunion with varus angulation.

Discussion

Recognizing the Problem and Situations at High Risk

Treatment of acute tibia fractures should be designed to maintain alignment, obtain union, and restore function while minimizing the risk of complications. Options include nonsurgical means, minimally invasive and invasive surgical means, or a combination thereof. Treatment decisions should be based on the character of the fracture, patient factors, and surgeon experience with the different available options.[2]

Closed reduction and cast immobilization are routinely effective for closed, isolated fractures of the tibia. Casts are effective in controlling angular and rotational alignment but are less effective in controlling translation and shortening. As a general rule, the amount of shortening that can be expected following nonsurgical treatment of tibia fractures is equal to that seen on initial radiographs. This is true even when initial reduction maneuvers reduce shortening. Also, nonunion develops in up to 6% of patients who are treated nonsurgically.[3-7]

Predisposing factors include high-energy fractures, segmental or highly comminuted fractures, open fractures, and fractures associated with vascular injury or infection.[8-11] Certain patient factors may also influence the development of nonunion, including chronic disease, poor nutritional status, a history of smoking, and type I diabetes.[12-15] The specific risk factors most relevant to nonsurgical treatment remain unclear because most studies examining this issue predominantly report on patients who have been treated surgically.

In the absence of fracture union, the diagnosis of delayed union can be made 4 to 6 months after tibial fracture, whereas the diagnosis of a nonunion is traditionally reserved until 6 to 8 months,[5,12] particularly if healing has not progressed over 3 months as seen on consecutive monthly radiographs.

Managing Aseptic Nonunion

Treatment of tibial nonunions should be designed to correct (1) axial and rotational malalignments and (2) limb-length discrepancy to allow functional restoration of the limb. Management options for an established nonunion include bracing, bone grafting, bone marrow injection, physical forces (eg, direct current, pulsed electromagnetic field, capacitive coupling, and ultrasound), and surgical repair (eg, intramedullary nails, plates and screws, external fixators) or a combination thereof.[1,13] Selection of one or more of these treatment options should depend on patient factors, the nonunion, and surgeon experience.

A rational approach to management of tibial nonunion begins with an understanding of the relative biologic capacity for fracture union. To this end, nonunions have been classified as vital or nonvital based on the presence or absence of callus and the radiographic appearance of the bone ends.[14] Nonunions with callus and without pencil tip-like ends are considered vital nonunions and include nonunions with large amounts of callus (hypertrophic nonunions) and those with less callus (oligotrophic). Those without callus and thin, pointed tips are considered nonvital or atrophic nonunions. Vital nonunions are believed to develop as a result of inadequate mechanical stability and therefore require stabilization for healing. Nonvital nonunions are believed to lack adequate blood supply and therefore require an improved biologic environment (eg, bone graft, improved soft-tissue envelope) and stabilization for healing to occur. Autologous iliac crest bone graft is the gold standard adjunct used to promote healing in nonvital nonunions. Historically, the bone graft is placed along the posterior aspect of the tibia through a posterolateral approach, as described by Hanson and associates[15] and others.[16] Additionally, "fish scaling" or "shingling" of the cortex proximal and distal to the nonunion site is performed in an effort to promote further healing.

Closed intramedullary (IM) nailing of tibial nonunions provides relative stability, early functional rehabilitation, and early weight bearing.[17-22] Compression across the nonunion site can be achieved when weight bearing is associated with dynamic nail insertion. Reaming, although shown in animal studies to disrupt the endosteal blood supply, may facilitate healing by providing local bone graft and a larger, more stable implant.[14] The indications for closed IM nailing of tibial shaft nonunions are (1) previously closed or prior Gustilo and Anderson type I or type II open tibial fractures, (2) fractures in the middle three fifths of the bone, or (3) when acute plating or nailing has failed. Reamed nailing of tibial fractures previously treated with an external fixator should be avoided when associated with a history of infection at the pin site.[21,23,24] When open take down of the nonunion is required (eg, medullary canal malalignment, severe deformity, or stiff hypertrophic nonunions), the benefit of closed nailing is diminished. In these cases, an alternative method should be considered. Unlike nailing of acute tibia fractures, nailing of tibial nonunions often requires hand reaming of the pseudarthrosis before the guidewire necessary for power reaming of the canal can be passed across the nonunion site. Reaming of the canal should be done without the tourniquet inflated to minimize the risk of thermal necrosis of the bone. In most cases, dynamic locking of the nail is necessary to provide compression at the nonunion site with weight bearing.[17-22]

Like IM nailing, open reduction and internal fixation (ORIF) with plates and screws provides stability and allows for early range of motion of adjacent joints. Advantages include application to virtually any location along the tibia and easier and more precise correction of any associated axial deformity. However, because plates are load-bearing devices, a period of protected weight bearing after fixation is required.[25] Other disadvantages of ORIF for nonunions include the increased soft-tissue dissection required; increased risk of infection, particularly in situations in which the skin has been previously compromised by injury or prior surgery; and the lack of rigid fixation in osteoporotic bone.

Ilizarov-type external fixators increasingly are being used to treat tibial nonunions, particularly for patients with associated bone loss, limb-length discrepancy, infected nonunions, and those needing multiplanar correction. The frames can be applied percutaneously with little blood loss and are stable enough to allow range of motion of the adjacent joints and

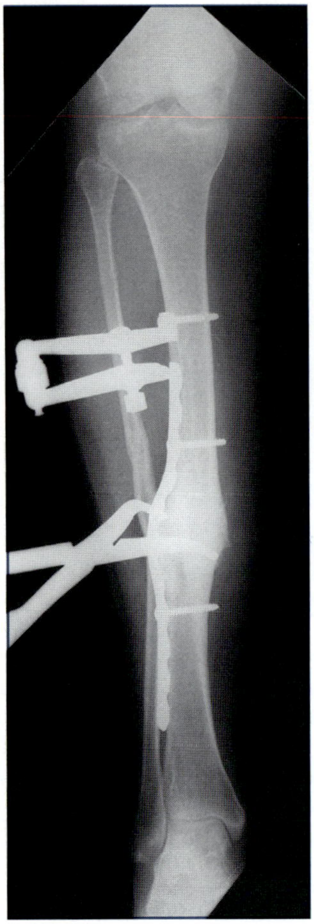

Figure 3 Intraoperative AP radiograph after correction of alignment with the use of an articulated tensioning device.

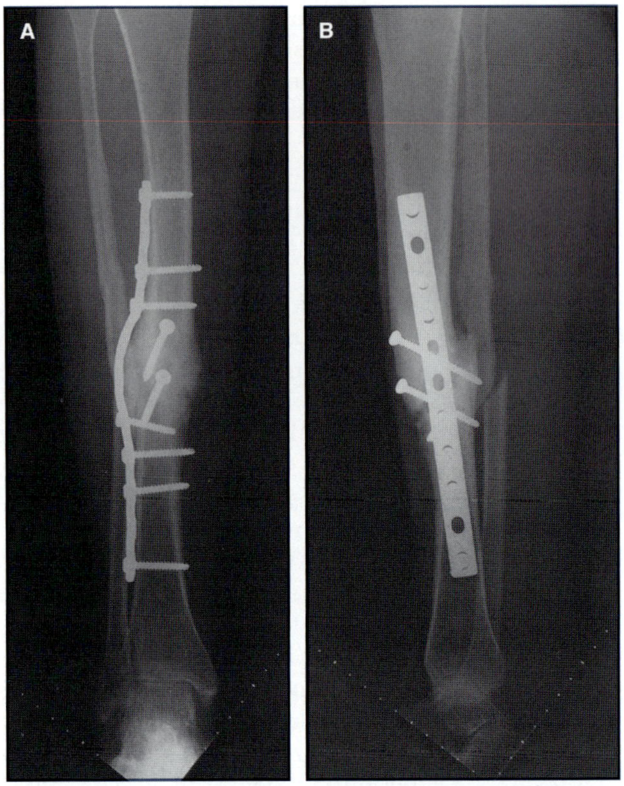

Figure 4 AP **(A)** and lateral **(B)** radiographs demonstrating healing of the nonunion and correction of the alignment.

early weight bearing. This technique is very demanding, however, and requires an experienced surgeon and a cooperative and compliant patient.

Preventing Failure of Nonunion Repair

Successful nonunion repair requires evaluation and proper treatment of both the local biologic environment and mechanical stability. Atrophic nonunions require augmentation of the biologic healing potential, usually with autologous bone graft, and adequate mechanical stability. The role for bone graft substitutes and growth factors is an area of expanding research, and these substances may soon obviate the need for autologous grafts. Oligotrophic nonunions have intermediate biologic capacity for healing. They require improved mechanical stability and consideration of biologic enhancement. Hypertrophic nonunions have adequate biologic healing capacity but lack mechanical stability. Rigid stabilization of these nonunions without bone graft is usually successful. In all cases of nonunion repair, restoring satisfactory limb alignment and preserving a viable local soft-tissue environment are necessary for consistent success.

Case Management and Outcome Summary

Three years after the injury, this fracture has the appearance of a hypertrophic nonunion with a healed fibula. Because of the presence of endosteal callus in both the proximal and distal fragment, closed IM nailing would have been difficult and would have necessitated opening of the nonunion site to clear a path for the reamer and guidewire. Therefore, ORIF with a plate and screws was selected as the method for repair.

The surgical technique included application of a pneumatic tourniquet to the proximal thigh. The leg was prepared and draped in the usual sterile fashion. The leg was elevated, exsanguinated with a compression bandage, and the tourniquet elevated to 300 mm Hg. A longitudinal lateral incision was made at the level of the tibial nonunion and carried down to the fibula. An oblique osteotomy of the fibula at the level of the tibial nonunion was performed and the wound irrigated and closed. A fibular osteotomy was felt beneficial to allow closer approximation of the tibial fragments during ORIF. A second longitudinal incision was made one-half fingerbreadth lateral to the tibial crest and centered over the nonunion. Dissection was carried through the subcutaneous tissue and medial to the anterior tibialis tendon. The nonunion site was identified and the lateral aspect of the tibial shaft exposed with the periosteum left attached to the bone. A large-fragment, narrow, limited contact-dynamic compression plate was contoured to the lateral tibial cortex and initially fixed to the distal fragment. Deformity correction and compression across the nonunion tie was accomplished with an articulating tension device (**Figure 3**). The plate was then secured with multiple additional bicortical screws. Fixation was augmented with two lag screws placed perpendicular to and across the nonunion site from anterior to posterior. The wound was irrigated and closed in layers over a drain.

Postoperatively, the patient was kept toe-touch weight bearing for 6 weeks then advanced to partial weight bearing; approximately 2½ months postoperatively, the patient was advanced to weight bearing as tolerated. The fracture healed without further complication (**Figure 4**) and the patient, for the first time in 3 years, was able to walk without pain and without assistive devices.

Strategies to Minimize Common Complications

If nonsurgical treatment is chosen, the fracture must be given adequate time to fully heal. Persistent pain and motion at the fracture site without bridging trabeculae at the fracture site or absence of progression of healing on three consecutive monthly radiographs are important indications of a nonunion. In this case, an obvious nonunion had developed. Two attempts at obtaining union with bone marrow aspiration and injection, an unproven method for nonunion repair, were unsuccessful. Treatment in this case, based upon the oligotrophic appearance of the nonunion, should have included augmentation of stability. Allowing nonunions to persist for prolonged periods of time makes subsequent treatment more difficult, less successful, and places a huge burden on patients and their families.

References

1. Connolly JF, Guse R, Tiedeman J, Dehne R: Autologous marrow injection as a substitute for operative grafting of tibial nonunions. *Clin Orthop* 1991:259-270.
2. Maurer DJ, Merkow RL, Gustilo RB: Infection after intramedullary nailing of severe open tibial fractures initially treated with external fixation. *J Bone Joint Surg Am* 1989;71:835-838.
3. Puno RM, Vaughan JJ, von Fraunhofer JA, et al: A method of determining the angular malalignments of the knee and ankle joints resulting from a tibial malunion. *Clin Orthop* 1987:213-219.
4. Puno RM, Vaughan JJ, Stetten ML, Johnson JR: Long-term effects of tibial angular malunion on the knee and ankle joints. *J Orthop Trauma* 1991;5:247-254.
5. Sarmiento A, Sobol PA, Sew Hoy AL, et al: Prefabricated functional braces for the treatment of fractures of the tibial diaphysis. *J Bone Joint Surg Am* 1984;66:1328-1339.
6. Suman RK: The management of tibial shaft fractures by early weight bearing in a patella tendon bearing cast: A comparative study. *J Trauma* 1977;17:97-107.
7. Trafton PG: Closed unstable fractures of the tibia. *Clin Orthop* 1988:58-67.
8. Jensen JS, Hansen FW, Johansen J: Tibial shaft fractures. A comparison of conservative treatment and internal fixation with conventional plates or AO compression plates. *Acta Orthop Scand* 1977;48:204-212.

9. Nicoll EA: Fractures of the tibial shaft. A survey of 705 cases. *J Bone Joint Surg Br* 1964;46:373-387.
10. Teitz CC, Carter DR, Frankel VH: Problems associated with tibial fractures with intact fibulae. *J Bone Joint Surg Am* 1980;62:770-776.
11. Waddell JP, Reardon GP: Complications of tibial shaft fractures. *Clin Orthop* 1983:173-178.
12. Johner R, Wruhs O: Classification of tibial shaft fractures and correlation with results after rigid internal fixation. *Clin Orthop* 1983:7-25.
13. Nelson FR, Brighton CT, Ryaby J, et al: Use of physical forces in bone healing. *J Am Acad Orthop Surg* 2003;11:344-354.
14. Schemitsch EH, Kowalski MJ, Swiontkowski MF, Harrington RM: Comparison of the effect of reamed and unreamed locked intramedullary nailing on blood flow in the callus and strength of union following fracture of the sheep tibia. *J Orthop Res* 1995;13:382-389.
15. Hanson LW, Eppright RH: Posterior bone-grafting of the tibia for non-union. *J Bone Joint Surg Am* 1966;48:27-43.
16. Simpson JM, Ebraheim NA, An HS, Jackson WT: Posterolateral bone graft of the tibia. *Clin Orthop* 1990:200-206.
17. Mayo KA, Benirschke SK: Treatment of tibial malunions and nonunions with reamed intramedullary nails. *Orthop Clin North Am* 1990;21:715-724.
18. Sledge SL, Johnson KD, Henley MB, Watson JT: Intramedullary nailing with reaming to treat nonunion of the tibia. *J Bone Joint Surg Am* 1989;71:1004-1019.
19. Templeman D, Thomas M, Varecka T, Kyle R: Exchange reamed intramedullary nailing for delayed union and nonunion of the tibia. *Clin Orthop* 1995:169-175.
20. Wiss DA, Johnson DL, Miao M: Compression plating for nonunion after failed external fixation of open tibial fractures. *J Bone Joint Surg Am* 1992;74:1279-1285.
21. Wiss DA, Stetson WB: Nonunion of the tibia treated with a reamed intramedullary nail. *J Orthop Trauma* 1994;8:189-194.
22. Wiss DA, Stetson WB: Tibial nonunion: Treatment alternatives. *J Am Acad Orthop Surg* 1996;4:249-257.
23. McGraw JM, Lim EV: Treatment of open tibial-shaft fractures. External fixation and secondary intramedullary nailing. *J Bone Joint Surg Am* 1988;70:900-911.
24. Tornqvist H: Tibia nonunions treated by interlocked nailing: Increased risk of infection after previous external fixation. *J Orthop Trauma* 1990;4:109-114.
25. Helfet DL, Jupiter JB, Gasser S: Indirect reduction and tension-band plating of tibial non-union with deformity. *J Bone Joint Surg Am* 1992;74:1286-1297.

Chapter 6

Infected Nonunion

Joseph Borelli, Jr, MD

Case Presentation

History

A 50-year-old man who was hit by a semi-tractor trailer while he was driving his motorcycle sustained bilateral midshaft femur fractures and Gustilo and Anderson type IIIB open right tibia and fibula fractures.

Initial Management

After resuscitation, the patient underwent bilateral retrograde femoral nailing, irrigation and débridement of the right leg, four compartment fasciotomies for an impending compartment syndrome, and reamed intramedullary (IM) nailing of the tibia. Subsequent irrigation and débridements of the right leg were performed 48 hours and 96 hours after the accident, and split-thickness skin grafts were applied to close the traumatic and fasciotomy wounds. Both femur fractures healed uneventfully.

Approximately 4 months after the accident, the patient had persistent pain in the right leg, radiographic evidence of a delayed union, and evidence of infection with increased pain, swelling, and erythema. Needle aspiration of the fracture site revealed purulent fluid that grew *Pseudomonas* and *Enterococcus* in culture. Based on these findings, oral antibiotics were prescribed, and the symptoms of infection resolved. Two and a half months later, the patient showed signs and symptoms of recurrent infection. Repeat needle aspiration showed similar culture results, and oral antibiotics were restarted. Soon afterward, a draining sinus developed along the medial aspect of the leg, and the patient was referred for definitive treatment.

Status of the Complication

History and physical examination suggested a chronically infected tibial nonunion. Radiographs (**Figure 1**) and results of laboratory tests, specifically elevated WBC, erythrocyte sedimentation rate (ESR) and C-reactive protein (CRP), confirmed the diagnosis. Each finding was consistent with an infected nonunion of the right tibia.

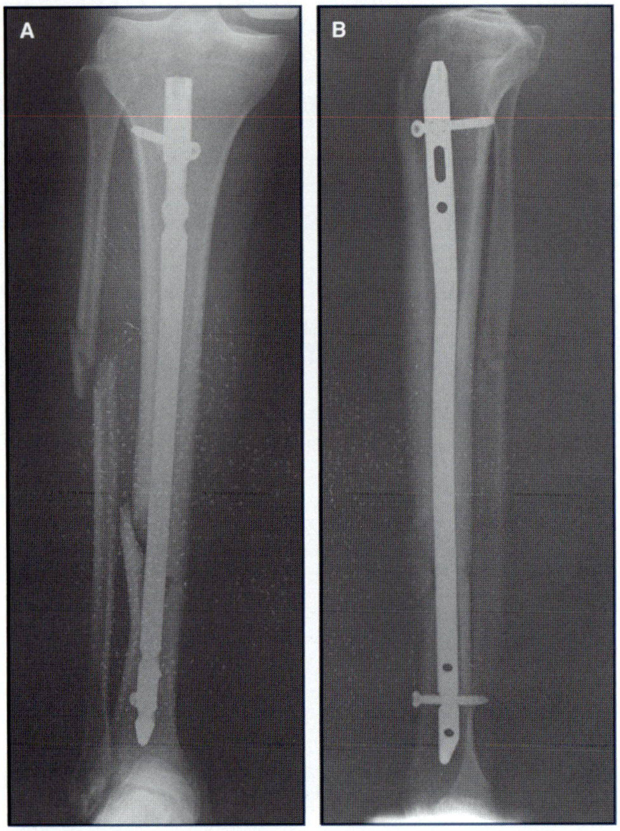

Figure 1 AP **(A)** and lateral **(B)** radiographs at the time the diagnosis of infected nonunion was made.

Discussion

Recognizing the Problem and Situations at High Risk

Open tibia fractures are typically the result of high-energy trauma and are often associated with fracture comminution and displacement, soft-tissue injury, and wound contamination. These conditions create an ideal environment for bacteria to proliferate. In the setting of diminished blood supply to the bone, it is not surprising that open tibia fractures are at increased risk for nonunion, deep infection, and infected nonunion.[1-6] The incidence of infection associated with open tibia fractures is considerable and reflects the severity of the injuries, including injury to the soft tissues and the degree of contamination.[1-3] In an effort to avoid these complications, initial treatment involves débridement of devitalized and contaminated tissues (including bone, muscle, fascia, and skin), cleansing of the wound, and stabilization of the fracture. To ensure complete removal of devitalized tissue, repeated irrigations and débridements should be performed at 24- to 48-hour intervals.[4,5] Recently, the use of antibiotic-impregnated bone cement beads placed about the traumatized bone and soft-tissue defects, in addition to systemic short-term antibiotics, has been advocated.[7-11] For open fractures with inadequate soft-tissue coverage, secondary closure with local or free vascularized musculocutaneous flaps should be performed within 5 to 7 days of the injury to decrease the risk of infection.[12-16]

The history and physical examination are key to making the diagnosis. Lotke[17] and others[18] emphasized that a history of open fracture, previous surgical intervention, pain and motion at the fracture site, and swelling suggest an associated bony infection even without drainage, systemic signs (fever is commonly absent) or symptoms of infection, or abnormal laboratory values. Certain laboratory studies can assist in the assessment and diagnosis of a musculoskeletal infection, specifically WBC (although this is commonly within normal limits), ESR, and CRP.[19-21] Unfortunately, these screening tests alone cannot be used to detect indolent infections because they lack specificity. Therefore, these indirect measures of infection have a good negative predictive value and are considered best for ruling out an infection.[20]

Plain radiographs and CT may assist in the diagnosis of infection, but because of complex posttraumatic changes in the bone, the often-present metallic internal fixation devices, and the presence of the nonunion, these studies generally are not diagnostic.[22] In fact, Tumeh and associates[23] reported that plain radiographs alone have a sensitivity of only 14% for the detection of bone infection. Technetium Tc 99m bone scans have been used in the past, but because of their high sensitivity and poor specificity for osseous inflammation, several common bony processes produce a positive result; therefore, this imaging modality cannot be used reliably to diagnose infection.[21] Gallium Ga 67 scans have been used in conjunction with technetium, but the combined accuracy rate is only 50% to 60%.[24,25] MRI is also of limited value in this situation because of the posttraumatic changes within the bone and soft tissues and the presence of metallic implants.[26-29]

Thus, diagnosing an infected nonunion, in the ab-

TABLE 1 May Classification System

Type	Description	Rehabilitation time
I	Intact tibia and fibula	6 to 12 weeks
II	Intact tibia and bone graft needed for support	3 to 6 months
III	Tibial defect ≤ 6 cm long and intact fibula	6 to 12 months
IV	Tibial defect > 6 cm long with intact fibula	12 to 18 months
V	Tibial defect > 6 cm long without a usable intact fibula	More than 18 months

sence of drainage, depends on the presence of multiple symptoms and signs, including the patient's history and physical examination, screening laboratory studies, radiographs, and a high index of suspicion. Definitive diagnosis can be made only by identifying bacteria either by light microscopy (Gram stain) or by culture of material from the suspected area of infection. Culture material can be obtained either by aspiration or biopsy at the time of débridement.

In 1989, May and associates[30] proposed a classification system for posttraumatic tibial shaft osteomyelitis (**Table 1**). This classification system focuses on the status of the tibia after soft-tissue and skeletal débridement. This system was reported to help determine the length of time needed for rehabilitation before a patient could ambulate without assistive aids.[31] Although this classification system helps estimate the time needed for rehabilitation and assists in the decision-making process, many patient factors, including age, health status, foot and ankle range of motion, neurovascular integrity, and motivation, have been shown to significantly effect outcomes.

The Cierny-Mader classification system for osteomyelitis is based on the anatomy of the bone infection and the overall physiology of the host.[32] Four types of osteomyelitis, specifically medullary, superficial, localized, and diffuse, are described in this system. The physiologic classes include the following: (1) A-Host, defined as a healthy host with a good immune system; (2) B-Host, defined as compromised locally (B^L) or systematically (B^S); and (3) C-Host, defined as patients who require suppression or no treatment, or in whom the treatment would be worse than the disease, or who are not surgical candidates. To identify the clinical stage, the type of osteomyelitis is combined with the physiologic class of the host[18,32] (**Table 2**).

TABLE 2 Cierny-Mader Classification System for Adult Osteomyelitis

Anatomic type	
I	Medullary osteomyelitis
II	Superficial osteomyelitis
III	Localized osteomyelitis
IV	Diffuse osteomyelitis
Physiologic class	
A-Host	Good immune system and delivery
B-Host	Compromised locally (B^L) or systematically (B^S)
C-Host	Requires suppressive or no treatment; minimal disability; treatment worse than the disease; not a surgical candidate
Clinical stage	
Type + Class = Clinical Stage	
Example: Stage IVB^S osteomyelitis—a diffuse lesion in a systematically compromised host	

Managing an Infected Nonunion

Treatment of an infected nonunion is influenced by its location, the integrity of the surrounding soft tissues, limb alignment and length, the condition of the host, as well as the needs and expectations of the patient. The approach to infected tibial nonunions begins with débridement of devitalized and infected tissues, followed by correction of alignment and stabilization of the nonunion, administration of culture-specific intravenous antibiotics, and creation of a viable soft-tissue envelope. The common goals of treatment are eradication of the infection and restoration of the soft-tissue envelope and bony integrity.

Débridement should include the sinus tract, the surrounding contaminated fibrous tissue, the nonunion site, and medullary canal. Débridement of the medullary canal is best carried out with flexible IM reamers that can be used through the nonunion site or through a portal of entry similar to that used for IM nails. Débridement should be accompanied by copious irrigation using a pulsatile irrigation system and approximately 9 L of saline solution. If the local soft tissues are fibrosed and scarred around the area of the draining sinus, excising this skin and the subcutaneous tissue should be considered. Subsequent flap coverage may be necessary to provide a healthy soft-tissue envelope around the nonunion to support bone healing and eradication of the infection. Such coverage may consist of a local cutaneous/fasciocutaneous rotational flap, local muscle flap and split-thickness skin graft, or free vascularized muscle flap and split-thickness skin graft.[33-36]

With the evolution of more resistant bacteria and the ever-increasing number of antibiotics available, infectious disease consultation may be advisable to provide guidance relative to the type and combinations of antibiotics, the route, and duration of treatment. Typically, intravenous antibiotics are administered only after material has been obtained for culture. The antibiotic regimen is then modified when the type and sensitivity of the organism(s) are identified. Other considerations in choosing the appropriate antibiotic are toxicity, frequency, and cost. The duration of antibiotic treatment is difficult to determine, but 4 to 6 weeks is common. The Cierny-Mader system offers guidelines for antibiotic administration based on the extent of disease and host type.[18] Depending on the antibiotics chosen, routine monitoring of peak and trough levels may be necessary to ensure therapeutic blood levels are maintained and to minimize the risk of toxic effects.[9,37-39]

Stabilizing a tibial nonunion is possible with IM nails, plates and screws, or external fixators. Stability is felt to help eradicate infection, improve patient comfort and mobility, and healing of the nonunion. Attempts are made to minimize the mass of implants within the infected area by using conventional half-pin or Ilizarov-type external fixators. Each method of stabilization has risks and benefits.[40,41] Ideally, once the infection is eradicated, the nonunion can be definitively treated in a planned, staged manner with either an IM nail, plates and screws, or an external fixator with or without bone graft. The bone graft can be placed directly into the nonunion site if adequate soft-tissue coverage is available; otherwise, a posterolateral bone graft technique can be used.[42-44] Bone graft materials can include autologous bone graft, allograft or synthetic bone graft substitutes, or a combination of all three. External or internal bone stimulators also can be used in an effort to promote healing.[45]

Preventing Infected Nonunion

Although infected nonunions cannot be prevented in each case, basic principles can be followed to decrease their likelihood. Open tibia fractures demand aggressive and thoughtful treatment. As soon as possible after injury, thorough irrigation and wound débridement are required to remove all devitalized and contaminated tissue. A "second look" done approximately 48 hours later is advisable to ensure that all devitalized tissue has been removed. Bony stability should be obtained and wound closure performed within 5 to 7 days of the injury. Early bone grafting (6 weeks) should be considered, particularly when bone loss has occurred. Antibiotics for 48 to 72 hours after definitive soft-tissue coverage has been obtained serves as an adjunct only and cannot take the place of wound cleansing.

Case Management and Outcome Summary

This patient had type III osteomyelitis according to the May classification (ie, tibial defect of < 6 cm with an intact fibula). According to the Cierny-Mader classification, the patient would be considered clinical stage IVA (ie, type IV, diffuse osteomyelitis with loss of bony stability before débridement, A-Host).

Once the diagnosis of an infected nonunion was made, the IM nail was removed and irrigation and débridement of the sinus tract, surrounding soft tissues, and the medullary canal was performed. The latter was repeated at 48 hours to ensure that all contaminated tissues and nonvital bone were removed. Tobramycin-impregnated cement beads were placed within the medullary canal and bony defect. Stabilization of the nonunion was obtained with a pinless external fixator in an effort to avoid further contamination of the medullary canal, although a traditional half-pin external fixator also could have been used (**Figure 2**). Culture-specific antibiotics were adminis-

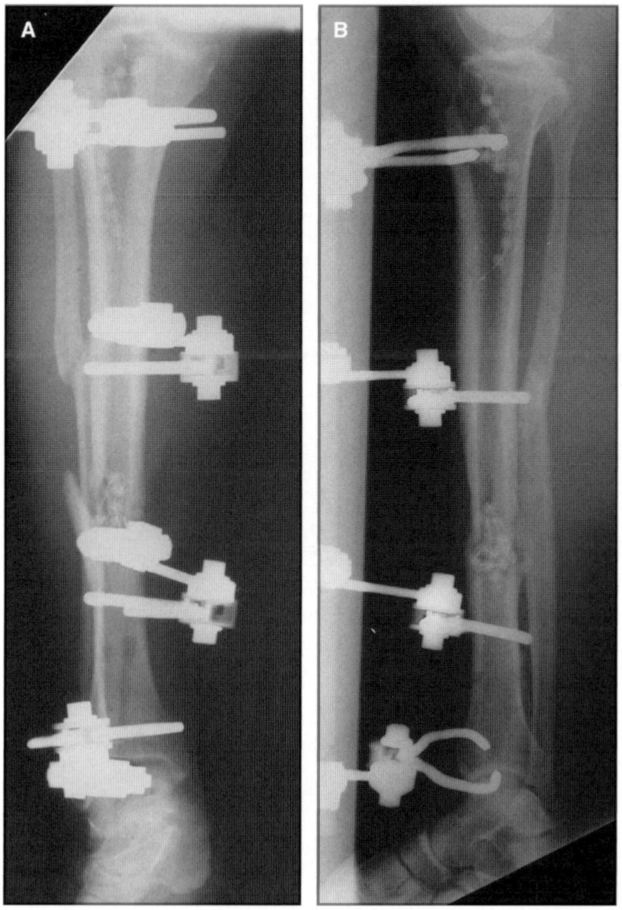

Figure 2 AP **(A)** and lateral **(B)** radiographs following removal of the IM nail, irrigation and débridement and application of a pinless external fixator. Note the antibiotic-impregnated beads at the infection site and within the medullary canal.

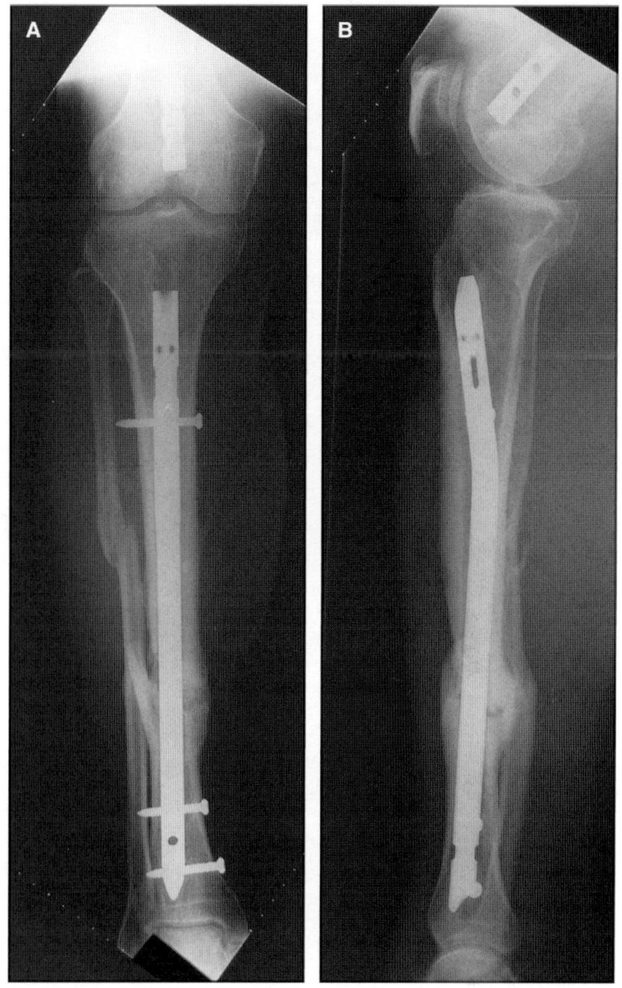

Figure 3 AP **(A)** and lateral **(B)** radiographs show healed fractures at the time of final follow-up after treatment with a reamed IM nail.

tered intravenously for 6 weeks at the direction of an infectious disease consultant.

Two weeks after completion of antibiotics, laboratory studies (ie, WBC, ESR, CRP) were repeated to assess the state of the infection. At this time, the patient had no pain in the area, the skin had healed, and there was no active drainage or palpable collections. Without clinical signs of continued infection and with normalization of the ESR and CRP, the external fixator was removed and a reamed tibial nail placed. Reamings from the medullary canal were collected, along with autologous bone graft obtained from the iliac crest, and placed at the nonunion site.[46,47] The IM nail was locked dynamically, and the patient allowed to bear weight as tolerated in the postoperative period. Complete bone healing occurred, and the patient is now pain free, has no swelling or other evidence of infection, and has returned to full employment (**Figure 3**).

The management of open tibia fractures is difficult and associated with an increased risk for complications. Initial management must be meticulous and include thorough irrigation and débridement of devitalized tissues, bony stabilization, and creation of a viable soft-tissue envelope. The diagnosis of an infected nonunion depends on the physical examination, laboratory studies, and radiographic images. Once the diagnosis is confirmed, treatment should be aggressive and include thorough irrigation and débridements of the infected area, administration of bacteria-specific antibiotics and restabilization of the bone.

Strategies to Minimize Common Complications

In the setting of a previously open tibia fracture, pain, erythema, and culture-positive material from the fracture site, combined with radiographic evidence of nonunion, confirmed the diagnosis in this case. Treatment of an infected nonunion with oral antibiotics alone is inadequate. An infected tibial nonunion should be considered a surgical condition. Removal of internal fixation devices, débridement of contaminated tissues and administration of culture-specific intravenous antibiotics is the standard of care. Recreating a viable soft-tissue envelope and restoring bony stability are critical subsequently in an effort to avoid further complications. Infected nonunions are potentially life-altering conditions and must be treated accordingly.

References

1. Blick SS, Brumback RJ, Lakatos R, et al: Early prophylactic bone grafting of high-energy tibial fractures. *Clin Orthop* 1989:21-41.
2. Caudle RJ, Stern PJ: Severe open fractures of the tibia. *J Bone Joint Surg Am* 1987;69:801-807.
3. Edwards CC, Simmons SC, Browner BD, Weigel MC: Severe open tibial fractures: Results treating 202 injuries with external fixation. *Clin Orthop* 1988:98-115.
4. Gustilo RB, Anderson JT: Prevention of infection in the treatment of one thousand and twenty-five open fractures of long bones: Retrospective and prospective analyses. *J Bone Joint Surg Am* 1976;58:453-458.
5. Gustilo RB, Mendoza RM, Williams DN: Problems in the management of type III (severe) open fractures: A new classification of type III open fractures. *J Trauma* 1984;24:742-746.
6. McGraw JM, Lim EV: Treatment of open tibial-shaft fractures. External fixation and secondary intramedullary nailing. *J Bone Joint Surg Am* 1988;70:900-911.
7. Bowyer GW, Cumberland N: Antibiotic release from impregnated pellets and beads. *J Trauma* 1994;36:331-335.
8. Buchholz HW, Elson RA, Heinert K: Antibiotic-loaded acrylic cement: Current concepts. *Clin Orthop* 1984:96-108.
9. Evans RP, Nelson CL: Gentamicin-impregnated polymethylmethacrylate beads compared with systemic antibiotic therapy in the treatment of chronic osteomyelitis. *Clin Orthop* 1993:37-42.
10. Miclau T, Dahners LE, Lindsey RW: In vitro pharmacokinetics of antibiotic release from locally implantable materials. *J Orthop Res* 1993;11:627-632.
11. Ostermann PA, Seligson D, Henry SL: Local antibiotic therapy for severe open fractures. A review of 1085 consecutive cases. *J Bone Joint Surg Br* 1995;77:93-97.
12. DeLong WG Jr, Born CT, Wei SY, et al: Aggressive treatment of 119 open fracture wounds. *J Trauma* 1999;46:1049-1054.
13. Gopal S, Majumder S, Batchelor AG, et al: Fix and flap: The radical orthopaedic and plastic treatment of severe open fractures of the tibia. *J Bone Joint Surg Br* 2000;82:959-966.
14. Gustilo RB, Merkow RL, Templeman D: The management of open fractures. *J Bone Joint Surg Am* 1990;72:299-304.
15. Templeman DC, Gulli B, Tsukayama DT, Gustilo RB: Update on the management of open fractures of the tibial shaft. *Clin Orthop* 1998:18-25.
16. Weitz-Marshall AD, Bosse MJ: Timing of closure of open fractures. *J Am Acad Orthop Surg* 2002;10:379-384.
17. Lotke PA: *Postoperative Infections in Orthopaedic Surgery*. Rosemont, IL, American Academy of Orthopaedic Surgeons, 1993.
18. Cierny G III, Mader JT, Penninck JJ: A clinical staging system for adult osteomyelitis. *Clin Orthop* 2003:7-24.
19. Covey DC, Albright JA: Clinical significance of the erythrocyte sedimentation rate in orthopaedic surgery. *J Bone Joint Surg Am* 1987;69:148-151.
20. Egol KA, Karunakar MA, Marroum MC, et al: Detection of indolent infection at the time of revision fracture surgery. *J Trauma* 2002;52:1198-1201.
21. Toh CL, Jupiter JB: The infected nonunion of the tibia. *Clin Orthop* 1995:176-191.
22. Bonakdar-pour A, Gaines VD: The radiology of osteomyelitis. *Orthop Clin North Am* 1983;14:21-37.
23. Tumeh SS, Aliabadi P, Weissman BN, McNeil BJ: Disease activity in osteomyelitis: Role of radiography. *Radiology* 1987;165:781-784.
24. Losbona R, Rosenthall L: Observations on the sequential use of 99mTc-phosphate complex and 67Ga imaging in osteomyelitis, cel-

lulitis, and septic arthritis. *Radiology* 1977;123:123-129.

25. Merkel KD, Brown ML, Dewanjee MK, Fitzgerald RH Jr: Comparison of indium-labeled-leukocyte imaging with sequential technetium-gallium scanning in the diagnosis of low-grade musculoskeletal sepsis. A prospective study. *J Bone Joint Surg Am* 1985;67:465-476.

26. Erdman WA, Tamburro F, Jayson HT, et al: Osteomyelitis: Characteristics and pitfalls of diagnosis with MR imaging. *Radiology* 1991;180:533-539.

27. Kaim A, Ledermann HP, Bongartz G, et al: Chronic post-traumatic osteomyelitis of the lower extremity: Comparison of magnetic resonance imaging and combined bone scintigraphy/immunoscintigraphy with radiolabelled monoclonal antigranulocyte antibodies. *Skeletal Radiol* 2000;29:378-386.

28. Totty WG: Radiographic evaluation of osteomyelitis using magnetic resonance imaging. *Orthop Rev* 1989;18:587-592.

29. Unger E, Moldofsky P, Gatenby R, et al: Diagnosis of osteomyelitis by MR imaging. *AJR Am J Roentgenol* 1988;150:605-610.

30. May JW Jr, Jupiter JB, Weiland AJ, Byrd HS: Clinical classification of post-traumatic tibial osteomyelitis. *J Bone Joint Surg Am* 1989;71:1422-1428.

31. Mader JT, Cripps MW, Calhoun JH: Adult posttraumatic osteomyelitis of the tibia. *Clin Orthop* 1999:14-21.

32. Cierny G III, Mader JT, Penninck JJ: A clinical staging system for adult osteomyelitis. *Contemp Orthop* 1985;10:17-37.

33. Anthony JP, Mathes SJ, Alpert BS: The muscle flap in the treatment of chronic lower extremity osteomyelitis: Results in patients over 5 years after treatment. *Plast Reconstr Surg* 1991;88:311-318.

34. Gayle LB, Lineaweaver WC, Oliva A, et al: Treatment of chronic osteomyelitis of the lower extremities with debridement and microvascular muscle transfer. *Clin Plast Surg* 1992;19:895-903.

35. Gordon L, Chiu EJ: Treatment of infected non-unions and segmental defects of the tibia with staged microvascular muscle transplantation and bone-grafting. *J Bone Joint Surg Am* 1988;70:377-386.

36. Patzakis MJ, Abdollahi K, Sherman R, et al: Treatment of chronic osteomyelitis with muscle flaps. *Orthop Clin North Am* 1993;24:505-509.

37. Calhoun JH, Henry SL, Anger DM, et al: The treatment of infected nonunions with gentamicin-polymethylmethacrylate antibiotic beads. *Clin Orthop* 1993:23-27.

38. McKee MD, Wild LM, Schemitsch EH, Waddell JP: The use of an antibiotic-impregnated, osteoconductive, bioabsorbable bone substitute in the treatment of infected long bone defects: early results of a prospective trial. *J Orthop Trauma* 2002;16:622-627.

39. Swiontkowski MF, Hanel DP, Vedder NB, Schwappach JR: A comparison of short- and long-term intravenous antibiotic therapy in the postoperative management of adult osteomyelitis. *J Bone Joint Surg Br* 1999;81:1046-1050.

40. Maurer DJ, Merkow RL, Gustilo RB: Infection after intramedullary nailing of severe open tibial fractures initially treated with external fixation. *J Bone Joint Surg Am* 1989;71:835-838.

41. Kocaoglu M, Eralp L, Sen C, et al: Management of stiff hypertrophic nonunions by distraction osteogenesis: A report of 16 cases. *J Orthop Trauma* 2003;17:543-548.

42. Borrelli J Jr, Prickett WD, Ricci WM: Treatment of nonunions and osseous defects with bone graft and calcium sulfate. *Clin Orthop* 2003:245-54.

43. Hanson LW, Eppright RH: Posterior bone-grafting of the tibia for non-union. *J Bone Joint Surg Am* 1966;48:27-43.

44. Simpson JM, Ebraheim NA, An HS, Jackson WT: Posterolateral bone graft of the tibia. *Clin Orthop* 1990:200-206.

45. Nelson FR, Brighton CT, Ryaby J, et al: Use of physical forces in bone healing. *J Am Acad Orthop Surg* 2003;11:344-354.

46. Sanders R, DiPasquale T: A technique for obtaining bone graft. *J Orthop Trauma* 1989;3:287-289.

47. Westrich GH, Geller DS, O'Malley MJ, et al: Anterior iliac crest bone graft harvesting using the corticocancellous reamer system. *J Orthop Trauma* 2001;15:500-506.

Chapter 7

Knee and Implant-related Pain after IM Nailing

William M. Ricci, MD

Case Presentation

History

A 35-year-old man who sustained closed midshaft tibia and fibula fractures as a result of an assault had extremity pain, obvious deformity, and could not bear weight on presentation at the emergency department. He has a history of smoking, alcohol, and drug abuse but no previous injuries to the injured extremity. Physical examination of the affected leg revealed swelling and deformity with ecchymosis and tenderness but no evidence of an acute compartment syndrome. Pulses were palpable and equal to the contralateral side, sensation was intact, the unaffected leg was normal, and there were no other injuries or abnormalities. Initial radiographs confirmed isolated closed midshaft tibia and fibula fractures (**Figure 1**).

Initial Management

The patient was splinted in the emergency department; the following day, he underwent intramedullary (IM) nailing through a midline incision with a patellar tendon splitting approach. The procedure was uncomplicated. Postoperatively, the patient was splinted for 1 week for comfort and thereafter began weight bearing as tolerated. Over the next several weeks, the pain and swelling at the level of the fracture gradually diminished. However, the patient noted increasing pain about the anterior knee and found that he could not kneel. Radiographs revealed progressive fracture healing with satisfactory alignment; however, the IM nail was noted to be prominent proximally (**Figure 2**).

Status of Complication

The patient has knee pain after IM nailing of a tibial shaft fracture.

Discussion

Recognizing the Problem and Situations at High Risk

Even though IM nailing is considered the gold standard for surgical treatment of tibial shaft fractures,[1] a significant incidence of knee and implant-related pain

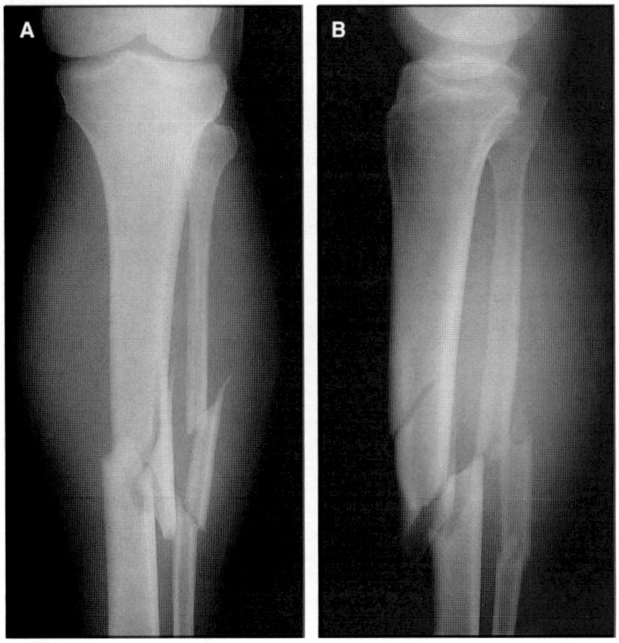

Figure 1 AP (**A**) and lateral (**B**) radiographs show midshaft tibia and fibula fractures.

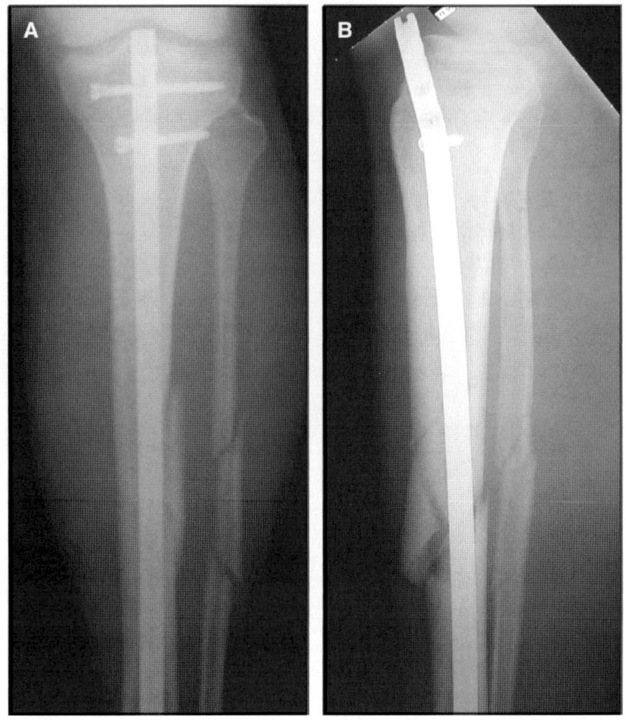

Figure 2 Postoperative AP (**A**) and lateral (**B**) radiographs show fracture healing with good alignment. Note the prominence of the nail, particularly on the lateral view.

has been reported.[2-7] Pain from proximal interlocking bolts that are too long can be the result of errors in surgical technique. Fluoroscopic AP radiographs obtained intraoperatively to confirm the length of screws can be misleading. The triangular shape of the proximal tibia can make screws of proper length appear shorter than the width of the tibia on an AP view. If the screw appears nearly the same width as the image on the AP view, it will undoubtedly be too long and cause hardware-related pain. Similarly, improper interpretation of fluoroscopic images can lead to prominent nail placement. Lateral radiographs centered at the nail's insertion site should be used to judge proper nail seating. A nail that appears to be properly seated in bone on an AP image can often be proved to be proud when evaluated on a true lateral radiograph (**Figure 3**).

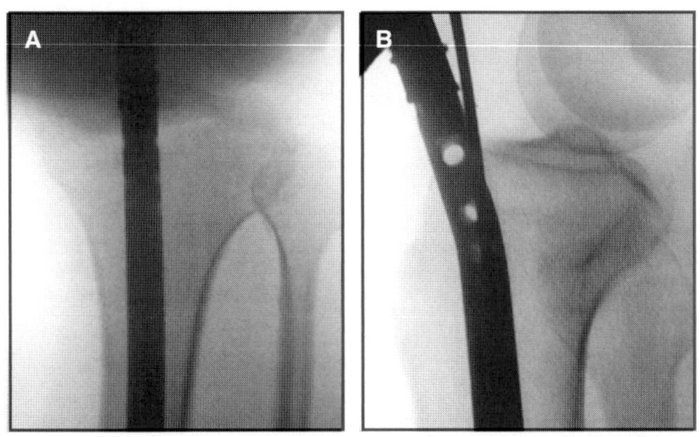

Figure 3 Fluoroscopic images of the IM nail insertion. **A,** On the AP image, the nail appears to be seated within the bone. **B,** On the lateral image, the nail is clearly proud.

Anterior knee pain is one of the most common long-term complications of tibial nailing.[2,5-9] Several authors[2,3,5,8,9] have reported that long-term knee pain after tibial nailing can be expected in approximately 55% of patients. Toivanen and associates[7] reported that 83% of their patients had postoperative knee pain. In the long term, knee pain can affect return to previous work in 10% of patients, interfere with activities of daily living and work in approximately 33%, affect ability to participate in sports in more than 50%, and cause difficulty kneeling in 75%.[3,8]

The cause and ways to prevent this complication remain unclear. Certainly, a nail that is left so prominent that it impinges on the patellar tendon will cause anterior knee pain. Nails that protrude to a lesser degree (so as not to impinge on the patellar tendon but protrude through the bone at the entry site) are not as clearly associated with knee pain.[5,7] Even when nails are properly seated beneath the cortex of the proximal tibia, a high incidence of chronic knee pain has been reported.[7]

The patellar tendon splitting approach also has been implicated as a causative factor. Retrospective studies have reported an increased association between chronic anterior knee pain and use of a transtendinous approach.[5,9] However, a retrospective review[4] and a recent prospective randomized study[11] found no difference in the incidence of knee pain in patients treated with either transtendinous or paratendinous approaches.

Unrecognized articular injury or meniscal damage has been suggested as another etiologic factor in chronic anterior knee pain after tibial nailing.[4] Damage to the infrapatellar nerve, surgically induced scar formation, and chondral injury from increased patellofemoral contact pressures during nailing also have been implicated.[7,10] Creating smaller surgical wounds, as with a percutaneous insertion technique, may decrease the incidence of knee pain.

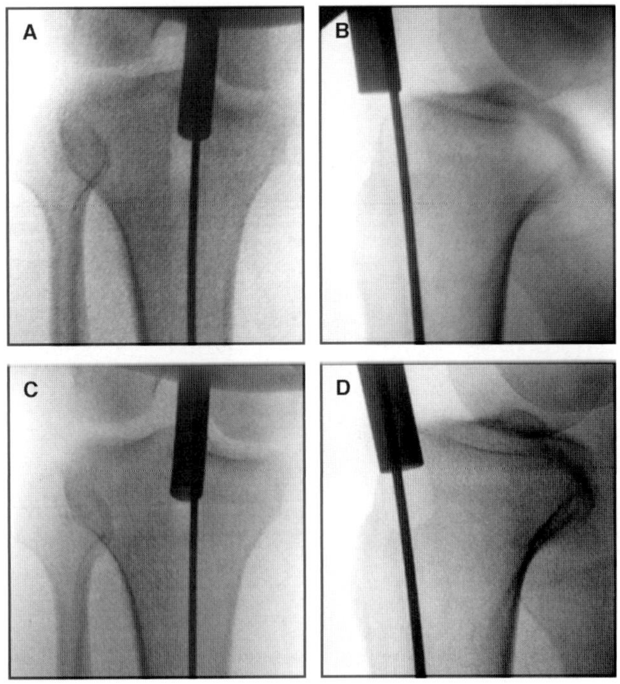

Figure 4 AP (**A**) and lateral (**B**) fluoroscopic images showing improper technique for measuring nail length. The depth gauge appears to be at the proper level on the AP view. However, the lateral view clearly shows that the depth gauge should be further inserted for correct length measurement. Proper technique is shown in **C** and **D**. The depth gauge is confirmed to be at the proper depth only on the lateral view.

Management and Prevention of Pain Related to Interlocking Screws

Prevention is the best management of implant-related pain. Meticulous surgical technique is important to ensure that all interlocking bolts are of appropriate length. Fluoroscopic images should not be used to judge the length of proximal interlocking bolts. Also, AP fluoroscopic images of the knee should not be used to measure appropriate nail length. Instead, lateral views are preferred to ensure that length is measured with the nail properly buried beneath the surface of the tibia (**Figure 4**). The shape of the proximal tibia must be considered when judging length of locking bolts. Even when a depth gauge is properly applied across the hole created for the interlocking bolt, the head of the screw often sinks into the soft metaphyseal bone at this level, leaving the tail of the screw proud. Both the head and the tail of the screw should be palpated intraoperatively to ensure that it is not prominent. If the screw is too long, it should be exchanged for a shorter one to avoid secondary surgical procedures.

Distal interlocking performed in a medial to lateral direction allows greater control of the amount of hardware (ie, the head of the screw) that protrudes through bone along the medial subcutaneous border. The tail of the screw at this level, even if slightly too long, is rarely symptomatic. The anterior tibial artery, deep peroneal nerve, and tibialis anterior tendon are at risk during AP distal interlocking.[11] These screws should be inserted through incisions large enough to allow clear visualization of these structures to prevent damaging them.

Management and Prevention of Knee Pain

Management of knee pain after tibial nailing is more controversial. Nail removal has been shown to reduce (by 27% to 45%) or eliminate (in 25% to 65% of patients) anterior knee pain.[2,5,9] However, up to 34% of patients have been found to have similar or worse knee pain after nail removal.[2,7,9] Medial parapatellar, lateral parapatellar, and patellar tendon splitting approaches have all been advocated for nail insertion.[2,5,7,9] A recent prospective randomized study found no difference in knee pain when comparing paratendinous and transtendinous approaches.[11]

I attempt to minimize incision length without compromising the safety of the patellar tendon. With blind percutaneous insertion, inadvertent injury to the patellar tendon is more likely. I prefer a mini open procedure with a 3-cm incision along the medial border of the patellar tendon, starting at the level of the inferior pole of the patella and extending distally. The incision is carried to the retinacular tissue, and a medial parapatellar retinacular incision is made under direct visualization. This approach allows adequate protection of the patellar tendon with tissue protectors during instrumentation of the tibia. Occasionally, especially for very proximal fractures, ensuring that the entry point is properly located (ie, centered with the long axis of the proximal fracture fragment) can be difficult or impossible through a medial parapatellar approach. In these instances, I use a patellar tendon splitting approach, again ensuring that the tendon is adequately protected during all instrumentation.

Case Management and Outcome Summary

In this patient's case, the IM nail was providing satisfactory support for the fracture, as demonstrated by progressive fracture healing. The degree of nail prominence, however, was causing injury to the patellar tendon. As a result, the nail could not be left in its original position. The nail was advanced into a more adequately buried position by removing the interlocking bolts, advancing the nail, and then replacing the interlocking bolts through new holes in the bone. At the time of operation, approximately one third of the patient's patellar tendon was eroded from impingement on the nail. The patient's knee pain greatly improved but did not completely abate. The fracture continued to union without further event.

Strategies to Minimize Common Complications

Meticulous attention to proper surgical technique is necessary to minimize the risk of implant-related pain.

References

1. Bone LB, Sucato D, Stegemann PM, Rohrbacher BJ: Displaced isolated fractures of the tibial shaft treated with either a cast or intramedullary nailing: An outcome analysis of matched pairs of patients. *J Bone Joint Surg Am* 1997;79:1336-1341.
2. Court-Brown CM, Gustilo T, Shaw AD: Knee pain after intramedullary tibial nailing: Its incidence, etiology, and outcome. *J Orthop Trauma* 1997;11:103-105.
3. Dogra AS, Ruiz AL, Marsh DR: Late outcome of isolated tibial fractures treated by intramedullary nailing: The correlation between disease-specific and generic outcome measures. *J Orthop Trauma* 2002;16:245-249.
4. Hernigou P, Cohen D: Proximal entry for intramedullary nailing of the tibia. The risk of unrecognised articular damage. *J Bone Joint Surg Br* 2000;82:33-41.
5. Keating JF, Orfaly R, O'Brien PJ: Knee pain after tibial nailing. *J Orthop Trauma* 1997;11:10-13.
6. Koval KJ, Clapper MF, Brumback RJ, et al: Complications of reamed intramedullary nailing of the tibia. *J Orthop Trauma* 1991;5:184-189.
7. Toivanen JA, Vaisto O, Kannus P, Latvala K, Honkonen SE, Jarvinen MJ: Anterior knee pain after intramedullary nailing of fractures of the tibial shaft. A prospective, randomized study comparing two different nail-insertion techniques. *J Bone Joint Surg Am* 2002;84:580-585.
8. Boyd KT, Tippett RJ, Moran CG: Anterior knee pain after intramedullary nailing of the tibia: Are knee function and work problems in the long term? *Proceedings of the Orthopaedic Trauma Association 2001 Annual Meeting*. Rosemont, IL, Orthopaedic Trauma Association, 2001, pp 53-54.
9. Orfaly R, Keating JE, O'Brien PJ:

Knee pain after tibial nailing: Does the entry point matter? *J Bone Joint Surg Br* 1995;77:976-977.

10. Devitt AT, Coughlan KA, Ward T, et al: Patellofemoral contact forces and pressures during intramedullary tibial nailing. *Int Orthop* 1998;22:92-96.

11. Bono C, Sirkin M, Sabatino C, Reilly MC: Neurovascular and tendinous damage with placement of anteroposterior distal locking bolts in the tibia. *Proceedings of the Orthopaedic Trauma Association 2001 Annual Meeting*. Rosemont, IL, Orthopaedic Trauma Association, 2001, pp 195-196.

Chapter 8

Malunion

Joseph Borrelli, Jr, MD

Case Presentation

History

A 37-year old man sustained closed isolated fractures of the fibula and distal right tibia in a motorcycle accident (**Figure 1**). Initial assessment revealed a well-developed, well-nourished, obese man with a history of type II diabetes mellitus.

Initial Management

After reduction, the patient was placed in a long leg cast and allowed toe-touch weight bearing. Radiographs at 4 weeks showed early callus formation at the fracture site, the cast was then converted to a patellar tendon-bearing cast, and the patient advanced to partial weight bearing. After further healing, he was placed in a walker boot and advanced to full weight bearing. Incomplete fracture healing, coupled with advancement of weight-bearing status, resulted in varus malunion of the tibia and fibular fractures. The patient was referred for further evaluation and management of the deformity.

Status of Complication

The patient experienced pain with ambulation along the lateral aspect of the foot and the medial aspect of his ankle and reported abnormal shoe wear and a nonhealing ulcer over the apex of the malunited fibula. Physical examination revealed an obvious varus deformity and an ulcer along the lateral aspect of the right leg. The patient's neurovascular status was intact, and he had full range of motion in both the knee and the ankle. Trials of several nonsteroidal anti-inflammatory drugs and orthotics were unsuccessful in relieving his pain.

AP and lateral radiographs of the tibia and fibula showed an 18° varus deformity of the tibia (**Figure 2**). Oblique radiographs, including 45° internal rotation and 45° external rotation views, confirmed that the apex of the deformity was solely within the coronal plane. Weight-bearing radiographs of the knee and ankle showed no degenerative arthritis in either joint.

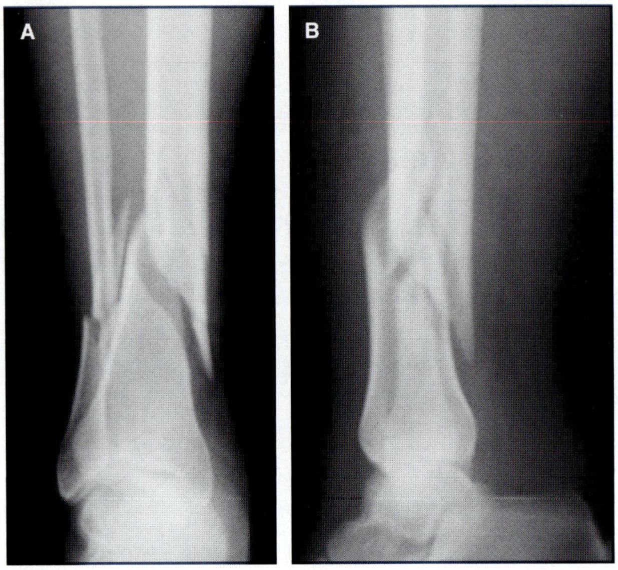

Figure 1 AP **(A)** and lateral **(B)** radiographs of the initial tibia and fibula fractures.

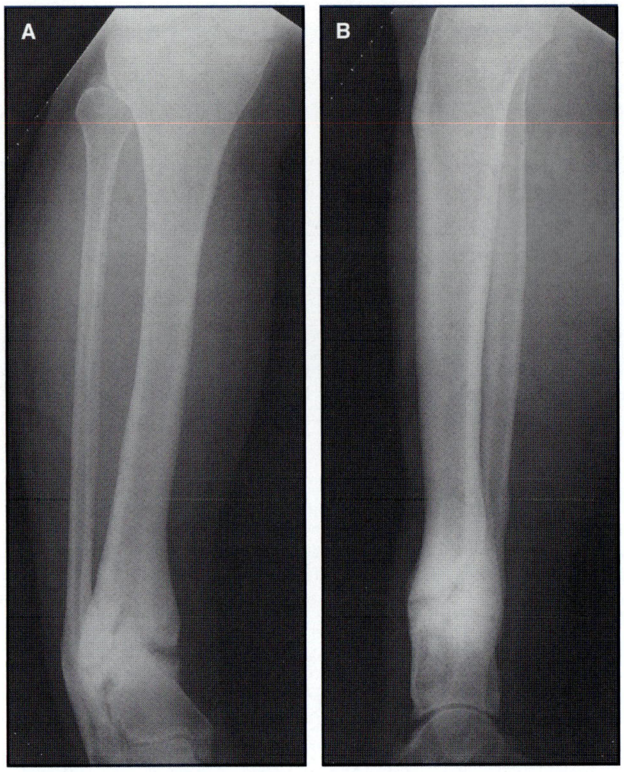

Figure 2 AP **(A)** and lateral **(B)** radiographs of the malunited distal one third tibia fracture with 18° varus deformity.

Discussion

Recognizing the Problem and Situations at High Risk

Malunion after fracture occurs because of an inability to obtain or maintain acceptable limb alignment. Risk factors include unstable fractures (eg, wide displacement of fracture fragments, diastasis between the tibia and fibula, less than 50% cortical contact between the major fracture fragments, and segmental fractures), fracture location, and host factors (large body habitus, noncompliance).[1] The consequences of tibial malunions are believed to depend on the degree of deformity, location of the deformity relative to adjacent joints, and the direction of the deformity.[2,3] Tibial malalignment has been shown to alter load transmission through the joints of the lower extremity, potentially causing chronic discomfort and possibly causing osteoarthritis (OA).[4-6] In vivo studies have shown cartilaginous changes consistent with OA in rabbits with 30° of tibial malalignment.[7] However, an absolute relationship between malunion and OA has not been established. In fact, several clinical studies have failed to demonstrate a definitive cause-and-effect relationship between tibial malunion and OA in the surrounding joints.[8-10]

Because tibial shaft fractures are the most common of all long bone fractures and because malunion may be associated with diminished outcomes, guidelines for acceptable reduction are necessary.[11] An acceptable alignment of the tibia is generally considered to be 5° of varus or valgus, 10° of procurvatum or recurvatum, 10° malrotation, and less than 1.5 cm of shortening.[2,3] Bostman[1] reported that if initial postreduction radiographs showed more than 50% translation between the principal fracture fragments, the chance of maintaining an acceptable reduction until healing was only 18%. Teitz and associates[12] reported that the likelihood of a nonunion or varus malunion was significantly increased in adult patients who have a tibia fracture with an intact fibula, if treated nonsurgically. Thus, indications for surgical management of closed tibia fractures include an inability to maintain an acceptable reduction, displacement of major fracture fragments of more than 50%, and tibia fractures with intact fibulas.

Successful nonsurgical management of closed tibial shaft fractures initially requires tolerance for long leg cast immobilization, protected weight bearing with use of assistive devices, and eventual early weight bearing in a fracture brace. Furthermore, these modalities require close monitoring, including frequent office visits, radiographs, and potentially frequent cast modifications. Although several large studies have reported that nonsurgical treatment of selected tibia fractures can be successful and the results satisfactory, recent studies have reported superior results with surgical stabilization.[13-17]

Managing Malunion

Nonsurgical treatment of tibial malunion includes activity modification, NSAIDs, and assistive devices. When nonsurgical measures are unsuccessful, surgical correction may be helpful, specifically osteotomy of the tibia and fibula with correction of alignment and stable fixation.[18] The goal of surgical treatment is to reestablish normal load transmission through the adjacent joints.[19] Preoperatively, the location and magnitude of the malalignment must be identified. Once alignment is restored, fixation options include open reduction and internal fixation with plates and screws or intramedullary (IM) nailing (**Figure 3**). Circular external fixators also can be used after corticotomy to obtain correction and stabilization. Plate osteosynthesis after osteotomy can be applied to malunion at any level of the tibia. This treatment modality corrects alignment and provides stable internal fixation obviates the need for postoperative immobilization. However, because plates are weight-bearing devices, the limb must be protected during healing by limited weight bearing.

Correction of tibial malalignment with an oblique osteotomy and internal fixation requires meticulous preoperative planning and is associated with some risks,[20] including infection, nonunion of the osteotomy, implant failure, recurrence of the deformity, and the need for additional surgery. Risk of neurovascular injury, which can also occur at the time of osteotomy, can be reduced by mobilizing the soft tissues around the tibia at the level of the proposed osteotomy and by placing retractors both medially and laterally to protect the soft tissues and neurovascular structures.

Preoperative radiographic assessment should include orthogonal radiographs of each tibia centered on the area of maximal deformity.[21,22] The osteotomy should be initiated with a thin saw blade, approximately 2 cm wide, and completed with a sharp, broad osteotome. Lateral fluoroscopic images should be used to help avoid penetration of the posterior cortex by the saw and further reduce the risk of neurovascular injury.

IM nailing following osteotomy is possible but can be difficult. Endosteal callus makes passing the guidewires and reamers difficult. In addition, if the medullary canal is reamed eccentrically, or if the tibial alignment is not held corrected during reaming, correction of the deformity tends to be suboptimal. However, the benefits of IM nailing include earlier weight bearing, promotion of callus formation, and secondary bone healing.[23]

Gradual correction of malalignment is also possible with distraction osteogenesis. This involves a corticotomy at the malunion site, application of an external frame, and gradual correction of the deformity.[24] Although this technique is less invasive than the others and can be used to correct all components of a malunion, including shortening, the design, application, and use of these frames is technically demanding and requires specialized training. Other disadvantages include prolonged use of external fixators, pin track infections, nonunions, and neurovascular injury during placement of the frame.

Preventing Malunion

Closed isolated tibia fractures that can be reduced and immobilized in an acceptable alignment can potentially be treated nonsurgically. However, frequent radiographs must be obtained to ensure that the fracture does not "drift" into an unacceptable alignment before healing. Generally, weekly radiographs are obtained during the first 4 to 6 weeks. Vigilance must be maintained once weight bearing is advanced because malalignment often develops at this time. If the fracture drifts into an unacceptable position, the problem must be addressed quickly to avoid potential long-term consequences of malunion. Closed cast manipulation (wedging), with or without anesthesia, can be

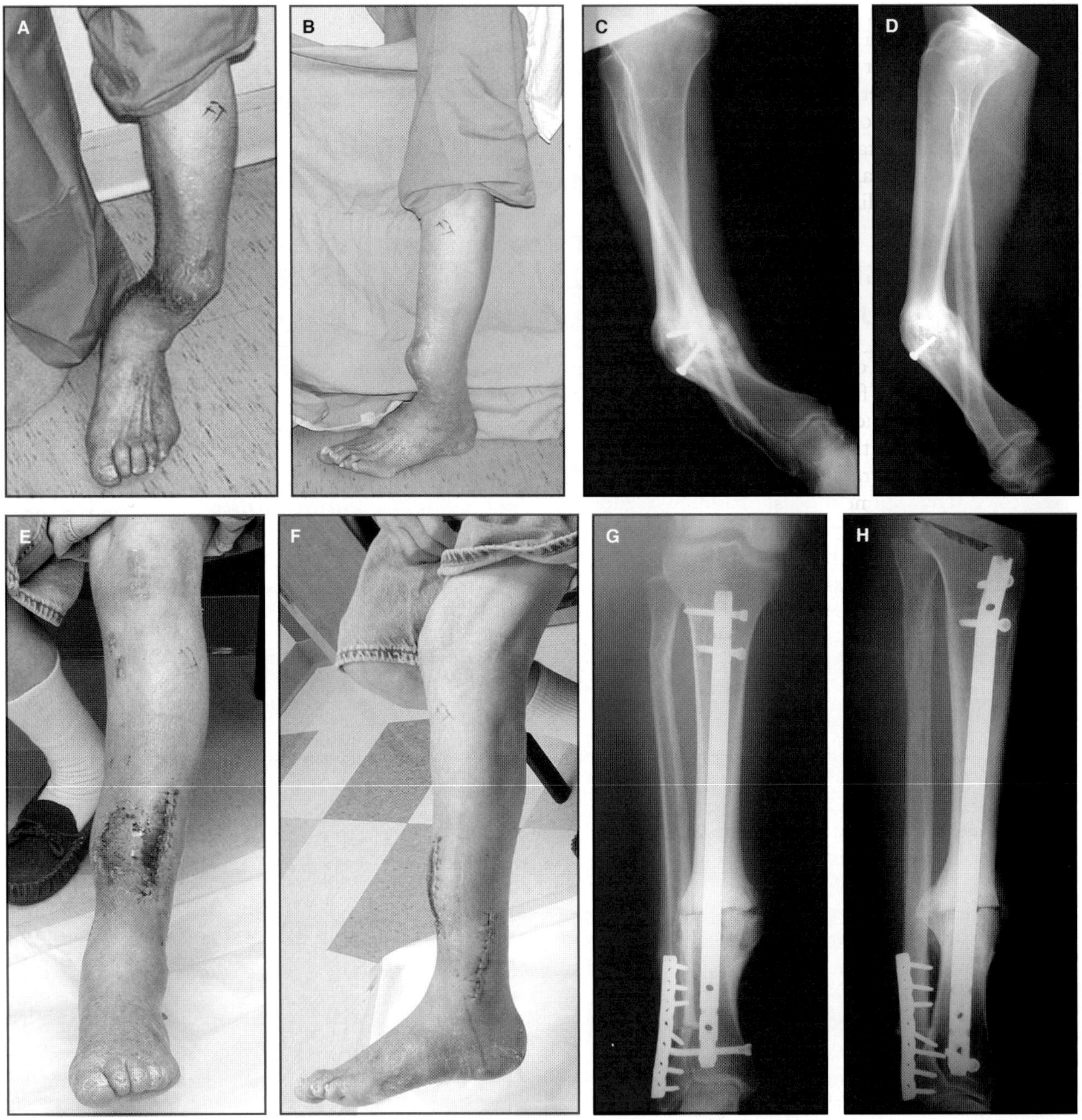

Figure 3 Correction of malunion with IM nailing. Clinical photographs **(A and B)** and AP **(C)** and lateral **(D)** radiographs of the preoperative deformity. Clinical photographs **(E and F)** and AP **(G)** and lateral **(H)** radiographs after surgical correction.

performed to realign the tibia. In many cases, however, surgical realignment and stabilization with plates and screws or IM nails are necessary.

The best treatment for tibial malunions is prevention. In most situations malunions can be prevented if the surgeon understands acceptable criteria for tibial alignment and remains vigilant regarding alignment during fracture healing.

Case Management and Outcome Summary

In this case, failure of nonsurgical management provided an indication for surgical correction. Preoperative evaluation included an assessment of (1) the soft-tissue coverage of the malunited area of the tibia, (2) ankle and knee range of motion, (3) limb length, and (4) tibial alignment. Assessment of tibial alignment was performed clinically and radiographically, with radiographs of the contralateral leg used for comparison and as a template for preoperative planning.[18,20,24,25]

Preoperative AP and lateral radiographs should be obtained with the x-ray beam centered over the area of maximum deformity. The deformity is directly measured by drawing two sets of lines and then measuring the angle at which they cross: the first set of lines includes one parallel with the tibial plateau and the other parallel with the ankle. The second set of lines includes lines perpendicular to each of the first. The deformity is measured as the acute angle between the second lines where they cross (**Figure 4**). Milner[26] noted however, that because of the slight "S" shape of the tibial shaft in many normal individuals, the actual "mechanical axis of the normal bone rarely passes down the middle of the medullary canal, making the conventional method of measuring the angulation of malunion potentially unreliable." Once the plane of maximal angulation has been determined on the orthogonal radiographs, the precise location and severity can be determined. Unless the plane of the deformity lies perfectly within one of the standard radiographic planes, the actual maximum deformity will be greater than that measured on either the AP or lateral radiograph. These angular measurements made on the AP and lateral radiographs can be used in a trigonometric formula or plotted onto graphs to

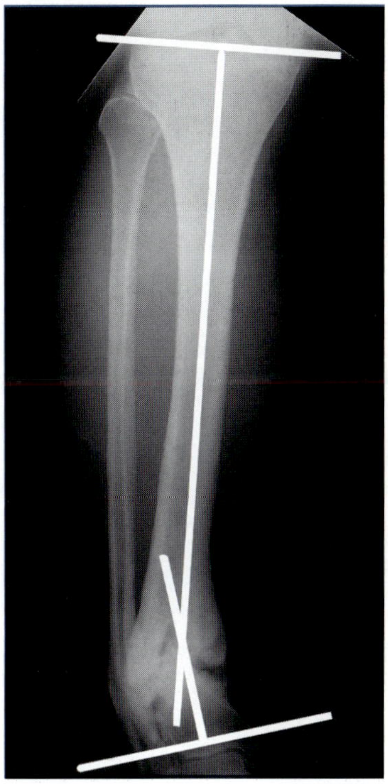

Figure 4 Measurement of the deformity. One set of lines is drawn parallel to the knee and ankle joints. A second set of lines is then drawn perpendicular to the first set. The angle between the second set of lines represents the magnitude of deformity.

determine the location and magnitude of the deformity.[21-22] Oblique radiographs parallel and perpendicular to the maximum deformity can also be obtained to reveal the actual magnitude and orientation of the deformity. Either of these methods will help in the selection of the appropriate plane for osteotomy.

In this case, preoperative radiographs confirmed an 18° malunion in the coronal plane (**Figure 4**). The preoperative plan called for an oblique osteotomy at the level of the deformity, perpendicular to the plane of the deformity. The technique, as described by Sanders and associates[18] was followed. In brief, both legs were prepped and draped in the usual sterile fashion. Initially, Schanz pins (4.5 or 5.0 mm) were placed at either end of the tibia. Proximally, the pin was placed parallel to the tibial plateau and distally parallel to the tibial plafond, both in the plane of the deformity (**Figure 5**, *A*). The leg was elevated and exsanguinated with a pressure bandage and the tourniquet elevated.

A straight anterior incision, one-half fingerbreadth lateral to the tibial crest was made over the deformed area. The malunion was identified; the adherent soft

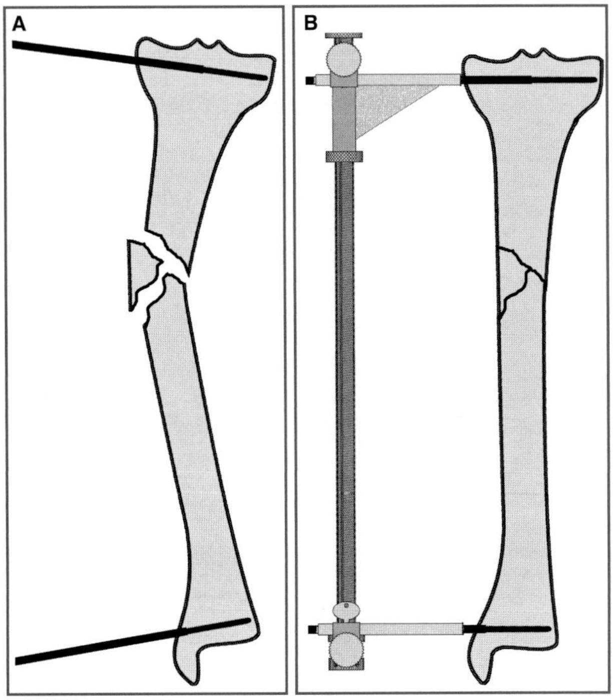

Figure 5 Use of the femoral distractor to obtain deformity correction. **A,** Two Schanz pins are placed, one each parallel to the knee and ankle joints. **B,** Adjustment of the femoral distractor until the Schanz pins are parallel provides correction.

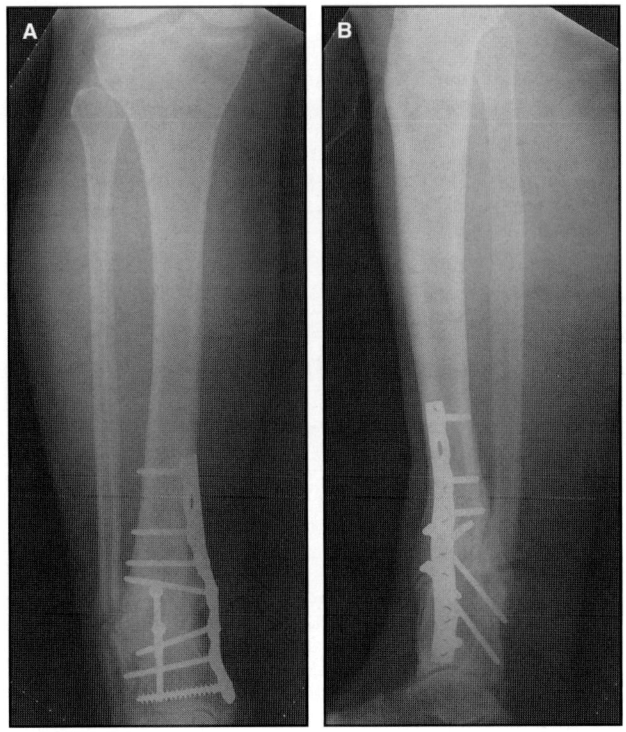

Figure 6 Postoperative AP **(A)** and lateral **(B)** radiographs after oblique osteotomy of the tibia and fibular malunion, fixation with plate and screws, and subsequent healing.

tissues were elevated circumferentially at the projected apex of the osteotomy, and Hohmann retractors were placed medially and laterally to protect the neurovascular structures. The tibial osteotomy was made as a single cut, obliquely, perpendicular to the plane of the maximal deformity. The saw was used to breach the posterior cortex, and an osteotome was used to complete the osteotomy. To allow correction, an oblique fibular osteotomy was made at the level of the tibial osteotomy site. Correction of the deformity was affected by lengthening of the femoral distractor until the Schanz pins were parallel (**Figure 5**, *B*). The osteotomy was stabilized with reduction forceps, and plain radiographs were taken to confirm the correction.

The alignment seen on these radiographs was compared to that of the uninjured side and to the preoperative plan. The legs were then compared clinically and because adequate correction had been confirmed both clinically and radiographically, the osteotomy was fixed with an anterior to posterior lag screw followed by a neutralization plate along the lateral or tension side of the tibia. Bony prominences of the previous malunion were removed with a saw and used for local bone graft after irrigation. The femoral distractor was removed, and the wound closed in layers over a drain.

Generally, short-term immobilization in a short leg splint is maintained for the initial 2 weeks postoperatively while the incisions heal. Patients are kept toe-touch weight bearing for 6 weeks and then advanced to partial weight bearing for 6 more weeks, provided radiographs are consistent with progressive healing. At 3 months, the patients are advanced to full weight bearing, and muscle strengthening is started. In this patient, the osteotomy healed, and he returned to work as a mechanic, with resolution of his ankle and knee pain and complete healing of the osteotomies and the soft tissues (**Figure 6**).

Strategies to Minimize Common Complications

In this case, advancement of weight bearing coupled with incomplete healing and insufficient frequency of follow-up examinations resulted in varus malunion of the tibia and fibular fractures. Whenever complete healing of tibia fractures that have been treated nonsurgically is in question, especially in patients at risk for delayed healing, weekly or biweekly follow-up coupled with cast manipulations and adjustment of weight-bearing status when indicated can help prevent the need for surgical intervention.

References

1. Bostman OM: Spiral fractures of the shaft of the tibia: Initial displacement and stability of reduction. *J Bone Joint Surg Br* 1986;68:462-466.
2. Greenwood DC, Muir KR, Doherty M, et al: Conservatively managed tibial shaft fractures in Nottingham, UK: Are pain, osteoarthritis, and disability long-term complications? *J Epidemiol Com Health* 1997;51:701-704.
3. van der Schoot DK, Den Outer AJ, Bode PJ, et al: Degenerative changes at the knee and ankle related to malunion of tibial fractures. 15-year follow-up of 88 patients. *J Bone Joint Surg Br* 1996;78:722-725.
4. Kristensen KD, Kiaer T, Blicher J: No arthrosis of the ankle 20 years after malaligned tibial-shaft fracture. *Acta Orthop Scand* 1989;60: 208-209.
5. McKellop HA, Sigholm G, Redfern FC, et al: The effect of simulated fracture-angulations of the tibia on cartilage pressures in the knee joint. *J Bone Joint Surg Am* 1991; 73:1382-1391.
6. Cierny G III, Mader JT, Penninck JJ: A clinical staging system for adult osteomyelitis. *Clin Orthop* 2003:7-24.
7. Wu DD, Burr DB, Boyd RD, Radin EL: Bone and cartilage changes following experimental varus or valgus tibial angulation. *J Orthop Res* 1990;8:572-585.
8. Kettelkamp DB, Hillberry BM, Murrish DE, Heck DA: Degenerative arthritis of the knee secondary to fracture malunion. *Clin Orthop* 1988:159-169.
9. Merchant TC, Dietz FR: Long-term follow-up after fractures of the tibial and fibular shafts. *J Bone Joint Surg Am* 1989;71:599-606.
10. Puno RM, Vaughan JJ, Stetten ML, Johnson JR: Long-term effects of tibial angular malunion on the knee and ankle joints. *J Orthop Trauma* 1991;5:247-254.
11. Bengner U, Ekbom T, Johnell O, Nilsson BE: Incidence of femoral and tibial shaft fractures. Epidemiology 1950-1983 in Malmo, Sweden. *Acta Orthop Scand* 1990; 61:251-254.
12. Teitz CC, Carter DR, Frankel VH: Problems associated with tibial fractures with intact fibulae. *J Bone Joint Surg Am* 1980;62:770-776.
13. Alho A, Benterud JG, Hogevold HE, et al: Comparison of functional bracing and locked intramedullary nailing in the treatment of displaced tibial shaft fractures. *Clin Orthop* 1992:243-250.
14. Bone LB, Sucato D, Stegemann PM, Rohrbacher BJ: Displaced isolated fractures of the tibial shaft treated with either a cast or intramedullary nailing. An outcome analysis of matched pairs of patients. *J Bone Joint Surg Am* 1997;79:1336-1341.
15. Hooper GJ, Keddell RG, Penny ID: Conservative management or closed nailing for tibial shaft fractures. A randomised prospective trial. *J Bone Joint Surg Br* 1991;73:83-85.
16. Littenberg B, Weinstein LP, McCarren M, et al: Closed fractures of the tibial shaft. A meta-analysis of three methods of treatment. *J Bone Joint Surg Am* 1998;80:174-183.
17. Sarmiento A: Displaced isolated fractures of the tibial shaft treated with either a cast or intramedullary nailing. An outcome analysis of matched pairs of patients (78-A: 1336-1341, Sept. 1997). *J Bone Joint Surg Am* 1998;80:1084-1085.
18. Sanders R, Anglen JO, Mark JB: Oblique osteotomy for the correction of tibial malunion. *J Bone Joint Surg Am* 1995;77:240-246.
19. Wade RH, New AM, Tselentakis G, et al: Malunion in the lower limb. A nomogram to predict the effects of osteotomy. *J Bone Joint Surg Br* 1999;81:312-316.
20. Mast JW: Preoperative planning in the surgical correction of tibial nonunions and malunions. *Clin Orthop* 1983:26-30.
21. Mast JW, Teitge RA, Gowda M: Preoperative planning for the treatment of nonunions and the correction of malunions of the long bones. *Orthop Clin North Am* 1990;21:693-714.
22. Ries M, O'Neill D: A method to determine the true angulation of

long bone deformity. *Clin Orthop* 1987:191-194.

23. Mayo KA, Benirschke SK: Treatment of tibial malunions and nonunions with reamed intramedullary nails. *Orthop Clin North Am* 1990;21:715-724.

24. Paley D, Chaudray M, Pirone AM, et al: Treatment of malunions and mal-nonunions of the femur and tibia by detailed preoperative planning and the Ilizarov techniques. *Orthop Clin North Am* 1990;21: 667-691.

25. Johnson EE: Multiplane correctional osteotomy of the tibia for diaphyseal malunion. *Clin Orthop* 1987:223-232.

26. Milner SA: A more accurate method of measurement of angulation after fractures of the tibia. *J Bone Joint Surg Br* 1997;79:972-974.

Index

Page numbers with *f* indicate figures
Page numbers with *t* indicate tables

A

B

C

D

E

F